Zen and The Art of Retirement

A Frugalista's Guide to Living an Untroubled Retirement in Troubled Times

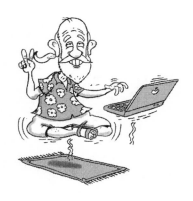

Louis D. Gonzales, Ph.D.

authorHOUSE®

AuthorHouse™
1663 Liberty Drive
Bloomington, IN 47403
www.authorhouse.com
Phone: 1-800-839-8640

First published by AuthorHouse 8/12/2009

ISBN: 978-1-4389-9631-8 (e)
ISBN: 978-1-4389-9630-1 (sc)

Printed in the United States of America
Bloomington, Indiana

This book is printed on acid-free paper.

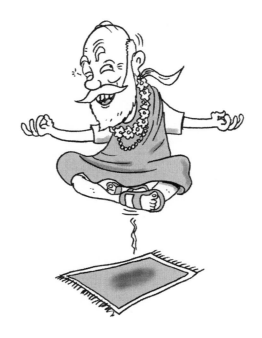

I consider it good Zen practice to share with others a piece of work one cannot hold onto anyway. Use this book however you want. Copy excerpts from it and share them. It's okay, really. The act of your sharing this goodwill with others will come back to you tenfold. I only ask that you at least buy the first copy, e-mail me for permission to use whatever pages or excerpts you need, and give me credit for my work.

Peace!

TABLE OF CONTENTS

ACKNOWLEDGEMENTS xi

THE BEGINNINGS xiii

WHAT IS THIS BOOK ABOUT? xv

FOUR UNIVERSAL TRUTHS xix

GOD'S MORTALITY SANDWICH 1
   Enjoy When You Can, Endure When You Must 2
   What A Long Strange Trip It's Been 3
   Dramatic Shift 5

WHAT IS ZEN ANYWAY? 9
   Zen: It Is What It Is 10
   Why Zen, Why Now? 10
   No Time Like The Present 11
   Unloading Excess Baggage 11

THE ZEN OF HUMOR 13
   Enlighten Up! 14
   Zen And The Benefits Of Retirement 14

FEARS, DOUBTS AND OTHER BUMMERS 19
   Mother Of All Bummers 19
   Shoulda, Woulda, Coulda 20
   Enough Already! 21

REALITY CHECK 23
   Denial Ain't Just A River In Egypt 24
   Through The Looking Glass 25

DEATH-PROOFING YOUR LIFE 29
   What Does Death-Proofing Mean Anyway? 30

The Zen Of Letting Go..30
Laying A Solid Foundation 31
Strategies For Death-Proofing Your Life.....................................32

THE "WE" GENERATION 37
Sixty: The New Forty (You Say?) 38

LIVING WITH PURPOSE 39
Sweet Mellissa...40
What's It All About?...41

ZEN AND THE ART OF RATIONAL SELF-INTEREST 43
The Darker Side Of Zen..43

STAY BUSY, DO LESS...45
The Zen Of Re-Wiring..46
What About Age Discrimination? 47
Look Up-To-Date 48

LIVING LA VIDA CHEAP 51
Untroubled Retirement In Troubled Times...................................51
Frugal: The New Cheap 52
Frugalista: The New Cheapskate..52

TOUGH TIMES CALL FOR DRASTIC MEASURES 55
The Mars And Venus Conflict 56
Women Are From Venus (And That's Not All) 57
Men are from Mars (And your point?)...58

LIVING THE FRUGALISTA LIFESTYLE..............................61
Ten Zen Habits of a Frugalista 61

ZEN AND THE ART OF BUDGETING 65
Running the Numbers...65

THE ZEN OF SHOPPING 69
Top twelve wastes of money and time:...75

THE ZEN OF EATING OUT A LA CHEAP 79

ZEN AND THE ART OF COOKING (AND SEX) 83
Tai Chi in the kitchen...83
The Zen of sharing 84

RECIPES OPEN THE DOOR 87
The Zen of ethnic cooking...87
It's all up to you now 89

THE ZEN OF ROMANCING ON-THE-CHEAP....................91

HOME IS WHERE THE ZEN IS 95
Declutter...96
Winterize...96
Buys in the 'hood 98
The Zen of an organized kitchen...99
The Zen of an organized bathroom 102

LIFE ON THE CHEAP 105

WHAT IF THIS FRUGALISTA LIFESTYLE CATCHES ON?..109

CREDIT WHERE CREDIT IS DUE..................................111

ABOUT THE AUTHOR...113

ACKNOWLEDGEMENTS

Have you ever wondered why books have "Acknowledgements" sections? Who reads them? Nobody I know. Sweating through a ton of research in preparation for this book, it finally dawned on me the point of these pages. Acknowledgement sections are a way for authors to pay back friendly debts to those they haven't had the pleasure of thanking in person. Now that this book is done, there are a few folks who come to mind.

A big thank you to Sister Holy Terror who, in the seventh grade, took great interest in a skinny, East Los Angeles kid and who "knuckled" him daily with her ruler until he learned how to diagram sentences properly.

I don't want to seem like I'm sucking up, but as long as we're acknowledging, I would like to give a shout-out to the collective works of Zen Masters Wayne W. Dyer, Richard Stallman, Alan Watts, Dean Sluyter and Melodie Beattie for their spiritual wisdom. Thanks also to frugalistas Ernie Zelinski, Robin Hearst, Julie Miller and Jeff Yeager for their practical (and sometimes bizarre) perspectives on enjoying life on-the-cheap. Their collective works helped keep the *frugalista* theme of this book within a Zen paradigm.

I am also deeply grateful for the kind and generous support of all who reviewed the book as it was being written, especially Merle, Briana and Gene who gave me feedback chapter by chapter and made it "flow" a lot better.

Too my kids: Save your money. Continue doing challenging and fun stuff.

THE BEGINNINGS

"Be patient and achieve all things.
Be impatient and achieve all things faster."

When I started the actual writing of this book, I wanted it to be a humorous, tongue-in-cheek take on retirement, free of deep moral and social messages. But after I got into the middle of it and began lining up all the topics I wanted to touch upon, other details kept coming at me like those annoying little pop-ups on a computer. Being just one year into retirement, I didn't know too much about it except for my own personal struggles when addressing the notion of suddenly being out of the loop and losing my identity as a wheeler-dealer, a rainmaker and clashing with some pretty bizarre experiences never encountered before retirement. I found myself struggling with the intermingled mental and spiritual aspects that kept crawling out of the woodwork like characters out of a Stephen King novel. The humorous material (my original goal) just kept drifting away making writing it a real challenge in itself. But I didn't want to stop and start over. I just let it take me where it wanted and see how it would play out...an unconscious process that in its own right created and maintained its own humor nonetheless. I have heard that the art of writing is about first   losing your inhibitions. And isn't that in itself Zen?

What follows is my crazy story; an unflinching analysis of my personal experiences and adjustments to retirement. It serves as a practical roadmap for the uncharted territory that lies ahead for all and soon-to-be retirees who may feel they are in need of some basic to-the-point direction, but who find themselves uncomfortable reading the same old, useless drivel cranked out by the Starbucks, laptop computer and cappuccino crowd who know very little about the 60-plus male psyche.

Now I'm not a cat-kicking, miserable old bastard...at least not yet, nor am I one who swears (not much anyway), but there are a few choice expletives sprinkled throughout this book that I've kept at a minimum. Why? Because this book may just have a shot at being displayed at Border Books or Walmart and I don't want to lose some good exposure just to get a chuckle out of you. Just know that the expletives are expressed for literary purposes only and are a result of channeling years of male cultural thought and emotion into one cool little book.

I invite you to make this book your constant companion in your new adventure. Use it as your primer, not only to teach you how to look within, but to help you fight for your freedom by laying out a plan that will allow you to live a practical and happy rest-of-your-life. Let's give our retirement adventure a try. Or as Miguel Cervantes' Don Quixote challenges us, "It is time to wield your lance and meet the source of your courage."

WHAT IS THIS BOOK ABOUT?

**"The only Zen you'll find on the mountain top
is the Zen you bring."**

Without getting too nitty gritty about some personal aspects of my life, let me just say that I'm a new male retiree about whom very little has been written or depicted outside of the movie *Grumpy Old Men,* which is precisely why I have prepared this book. It is for any man who may be in the throes of retirement and at a loss as to what to do next with all those hours of extra time in a shrinking economy and on a limited budget. It integrates some aspects of Zen philosophy with retirement guidance on how one can begin to embrace this new life-phase and still be able to live a fun and frugal lifestyle. Though it has been written from a male's perspective, I have to say that I have been pleasantly surprised by the number of female reviewers who read it and came to view it as an enjoyable guidebook for them as well. Which only proves what Zen teaches: We are all made from the same substances and deep down nothing is either male or female.

Three months into my retirement, I found myself on my deck reading in bewilderment about the downward spiraling economy and how social security benefits are going to run out by 2030. I thought, "Damn! How the hell do they do it?" Retirees, I mean. How was I going to do it? It didn't take long to realize that maybe I had not properly prepared creatively for what retirement gurus refer to as the "second life." I thought I had done all my homework. Let's see.

The web research has been very clear. Anyone making a retirement consideration should have: a good financial plan (the small nest egg I had laid seemed sufficient); a positive outlook (no problem there); a good and consistent exercise program (shivering through four winter months in Minnesota does not count as an aerobic exercise); and a wad of cash stashed away in the basement to pay for expensive vacation condos in winter and those long, boring cruiseliner trips to nowhere. I had begun to think that maybe perpetual idleness sucked (to quote my kids), that maybe all those retirement talks back at the office were a lot of overrated nonsense.

I also realized that retirement wasn't just about laying out a good financial plan. Though, that's always first on people's minds. I now suddenly had over forty hours of extra time to do whatever I wanted to, but didn't have a plan. Being a type "A" workaholic and with no real hobbies or productive activities to carry me through, it quickly began to sink in that I couldn't mentally survive retirement if my only creative challenges were going to consist of more fishing, more golf, weekly trips to the casino and moving plants from one end of the yard to the other. Retirement felt like someone had slammed the gates in my face and I was left on the outside looking in.

Frustrated from reading my limit of recycled, new-age theories from those god-awful self-help books and three brief sessions of *transition counseling* with a thirty-something who kept trying to talk me into giving myself permission to *embrace* my experience, I quickly discovered that very little was out there for guys who are on a limited income and facing a daunting new stage in life. The books that were available about surviving a challenging economy and living a frugal lifestyle were mostly written by women, for women and for college kids. Somewhat helpful, but limiting nonetheless. It seemed easier to find information on bomb-making then on issues relating to male retirement. Depressing, to say the least. But then again, aren't depressed people usually the ones with the best grasp of the situation thus better able to write about it?" So I decided to ignore the experts and write my own stuff from my own experiences and see where it would take me. Zen teaches that expert guidance only saves time. The heavy work is still really up to you.

Several of the retirement philosophies and the over one hundred frugal tips I have picked up along the way, came from my own fall-down-push-myself-up involvement with having to adjust to a strange, new life-phase. I've made wall-to-wall mistakes in the process, but have had the *cojones* to document and share them with other men who perhaps did not plan for an unexpected retirement and are now suddenly realizing, as I did, that they are suddenly on their own facing a soaring cost of living, an economy that is circling the toilet bowl and not a clue about how to budget, shop, and cut corners.

Maybe that's how you got to this section of the bookstore as you've suddenly realized that you weren't that great of a financial planner in the first place, and are now seeing your nest egg go *pffshshhhh* like a leaky air mattress and you can't get a bailout loan from the fat cats in Washington. I feel your pain. Relax. Take a deep breath. I have the answers you seek.

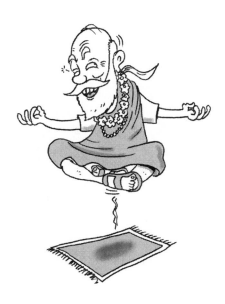

FOUR UNIVERSAL TRUTHS

"When there are no unnecessary thoughts in your mind every day is a good day."

I'm guessing you're like me and like to cut to the chase: "Where are the frugal tips dammit? Why do I have to read all this Zen stuff first?" Slow down... find your center. The simple thing would have been for me to print you a long list of frugal tips for you to select. But if that is all I do, you would be missing the whole point. Retirement is more than having sufficient financial resources (libraries are full of such topics) to live out a good life. Retirement is also about having a healthy attitude about where you are at this moment in life and taking stock of those things that are now important to you.

This book requires that you pour yourself a long drink, relax and take it all in. It has been divided into four universal truths... and for good reason. Because we are living in a busy, complicated and ever-changing world, each truth addresses a unique aspect of living a happier and stress-free retirement lifestyle. It is not a stand-alone book that one can just open up and pick out what one likes. One truth cannot exist without the other. So it must be read in its entirety in order for it to make greater sense.

Truth #1: *Stuff happens*...then you move on. This is a great cliché for accepting reality and is a big part of Zen thinking. Life is full of imperfections. Things change, so expect surprises. Everyone must prepare for the unexpected emotional, physical and financial realities of retirement in these trying times. Don't waste time over-analyzing things you can't explain, change or control. In other words, stop sweating the small stuff. You're retired now. Everything should be small stuff. I like to say, if life starts throwing lemons at you, grab the tequila. It's now time to begin letting go of people and things that don't nurture your philosophy, needs and spirit. Start investing in yourself.

Truth #2: *Age happens.* Think of yourself as young and you will be. Don't believe it? Anyone who has taken basic science 101 knows that "thinking" is a natural involuntary reflex. Like an ocean's ecosystem, the thinking process floats around and goes where it wants to. But you can learn to control what you think about and when. A healthy mental state is just as important as a healthy physical state when you begin to age. I like to say that a healthy mental state creates energy. That energy then creates more energy. And when that energy is channeled into thinking young, you'll never need to feel old again. Never underestimate the power and energy of thought.

Truth #3: *Laughter is good medicine.* Life is short and you'll never get out alive. There isn't one shred of evidence that life is supposed to be serious. Some days you're the dog, other days you're the fire hydrant. Stuff just happens. But by maintaining a positive attitude and laughing more, you will begin to death-proof your life. To quote Quincy Jones (musician/author): "A big laugh is a really loud noise from the soul saying, 'Ain't that the truth.'"

Truth #4: *A dream without a plan is a nightmare.* Retirement planning is just not about finances. The sudden (unstructured) freedom associated with retirement can also be just as daunting as financial considerations. But by visualizing, personalizing and reframing a retirement future for yourself that focuses more on the personal, social, health, and lifestyle considerations you expect to have, you can better prioritize those things that are important to you and give your dreams substance. I say personalizing your dreams because through personalization comes ownership and if you own your dreams, then no one can take them away from you. If you know why your dreams are important to you, it will put power behind figuring out how to achieve them. Don't let anyone drive a wedge between you and your dreams. Zen teaches that the key to successful aging is to pay as little attention to it as possible.

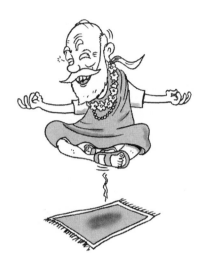

GOD'S MORTALITY SANDWICH

"Be here and now. Be someplace else later."

Every book has a story behind it and I thought you might be interested in the story behind this one. Without getting too invested in the nitty gritty details of a particular moment in my life, let me just briefly disclose why I retired earlier than I had expected.

People have a great variety of reasons to opt for retirement. One of the most common ones seems to be the one forced upon us through someone elses company policy. (Now that time doesn't matter, they present you with a cheap watch.) Another is financial; the desire to afford and enjoy a life of perpetual leisure. (Nice work if you can get it.) A third common reason is the desire for freedom...to take your nest egg and give the day-to-day hustle the finger and try your hand at a home business. (Fun, but risky.) A fourth and final reason is the one where God hands you a *mortality sandwich* (an unexpected event that suddenly grabs your attention). In my case, it was a minor stroke followed months later by A-fib, a medical term for atrial fibrillation meaning your heart is beating irregularly and you could die. I can still recall being slumped in a chair, staring at the designs on the rug hearing the sirens getting louder by the second and flashing a helpless grin while mumbling, "Damn, I've maxed out my mileage. My ride's here."

Enjoy When You Can, Endure When You Must

This is the endure part. Strapped in a gurney, all I could do was stare at the white roof of the ambulance, which in my disoriented mind resembled a wide screen TV that kept my eyes frozen at flashbacks of my life. (If you've ever wondered if this really happens, it does, really.) At a weak attempt to hide the one tear that found its way out of my left eye, I thought, "Crap, is this all there is?" At the hospital, I was given two options: 1) Take drugs that slow down the heart rate and maybe the rhythm will return to normal, maybe... 2) Take a ride on the electrical conversion machine where they stop your heart for five seconds (no choir, no angels, no white light), followed by placing paddles on your chest and then it's "clear, clear" then bzzzzzsssttt! It was God's tough-love way of saying slow down, listen to your body (and a lower-than-whale-shit moment in my life). If you ever start to get this weird feeling in your chest the next time you get up early to pee, you might just want to check it out.

Up until that unpleasant incident, the world and all its challenges had convinced me that what I had been longing for (retirement) was just too far off to reach. I kept the goal on the back burner, you know, maybe next year. Initially this plan of delayed gratification seemed rational and intelligent to me. But God's early warning got my attention and put me closer to retirement whether I was ready for it or not. My first epiphany was an awareness that life is short. I mean, when God hands you a mortality sandwich, you don't send it back. ("Come back later God, I need a little more time with the menu.") You must eat it, meaning you have to chew it, process it and swallow some hard realities. I had to drop everything, regroup and sort stuff out. That took about six months. Sitting through several weeks of recovery my dilemma was figuring how not to become paralyzed in self-pity and how to channel the awareness that life is short into something positive once I get out of the rat race (and learn to survive on less cheese).

I kept mulling over what I would enjoy with my leisure time and how I would earn enough WAM (Walking Around Money) to supplement my pension and Social Security and live out a stress-free life, while all the time arriving at the same conclusion: writing and working with young people with educational needs. I always thought I was a better-than-average writer. And I could always dust off my teaching license and volunteer or teach part time. Still, my critics kept reminding me that volunteering and writing may be great for the spirit, but not the wallet. But I'm not one that's easily swayed by critics (two clowns don't make a circus). For some strange reason, today, earning a bundle of money is not that important to me. Time is no longer so much about money. Time is a gift given to me to do those things I love. But I'm no dummy either. Money is important to the extent that one needs resources to survive, naturally. It's rough out there. I'm only talking about the importance of maintaining a frugal mindset while still having enough resources to enjoy every aspect of life. I'll talk more about this later.

What A Long Strange Trip It's Been

This chapter would have been better titled: True confessions. Two weeks after a brief recovery, I submitted my retirement letter to my board of directors, cleaned out my office and tossed my laptop into my car. As I drove off, I cranked up the car stereo as always and heard the Grateful Dead's ironic lament, *"...lately it occurs to me, what a long strange trip it's been."* That verse from *Truckin'* was the intuitive sign that removed all doubts...my second epiphany. I had made the right choice. Unbeknown to me, there were still greater choices to be made further on down the road.

Although my career in education found me working with some pretty spectacular people, I am saddened by the fact that my life had been focused on the pragmatic, superficial side, at times biting off more than I could chew just to strengthen my ego and fatten my wallet. It was always about maintaining my external identity (*what* I was) and ignoring my internal self (*who* I was) and all the time spinning my wheels. But don't get down on me for that. Having been known as an unconventional troubleshooter, an educational visionary and, at times, a bit unorthodox (I got things done), I nonetheless managed to make some cool power plays and come up with some creative solutions to some very sticky urban, educational challenges. If something didn't work for kids, I would introduce legislation to change it. My board chair always quipped that if I were to die and go to hell, I'd soon figure out a way to air condition it.

It was during this period that many innovations were being created in urban education and many greater opportunities were created for a lot of young inner city kids. Sure, I received recognition for my efforts: inscribed coffee mugs, plaques, pictures of me with a government official I didn't even know, a designated parking spot and, oh yes, a knockoff Rolex. I had achieved everything I wanted in life...material possessions, a great family, a big house near Lake Minnetonka (a place where people live well and kids test well) and my black-on-black SUV. Still, I felt unfulfilled. I was all about making it and not about making it matter. It seemed that I had grown vertically, but not horizontally.

Still, I have no real regrets. I have learned two things in retirement: One is that our purpose on earth is to simply experience life and to accept and make the most of it, and two, that one is imperfect and we all make mistakes and these mistakes are a part of growing. On occasion, we find ourselves taking two steps back. And that's okay. Sometimes it's a necessary part of moving forward.

You see, our growth is not one dimensional. We grow partially, always changing with circumstances in our lives. We grow unevenly, at different times and according to different experiences. We grow unexpectedly with some experiences catapulting us forward and others holding us back. Still others have us fixed in the present. But they all mingle together to make us the persons that we are.

An ancient proverb says, "The best time to plant a tree was twenty years ago. The second best time is now." Meaning that it's never too late to revisit and renew priorities. I have now decided to slow down the merry-go-round in my head and start anew, to strip away the layers of obsolete information and ingrained biases that had been taught in the past. I now sit in front of this computer sipping a (lukewarm) cup of coffee, feeling a little more introspective, no longer a hedonistic follower of schemes, but instead a bloodshot-eyed freelance writer who finds himself leaning a lot closer than natural into a computer screen for a better view at those obscure fonts, and who chooses to work just three days per week with some pretty awesome special needs kids, not for the money, but just because.

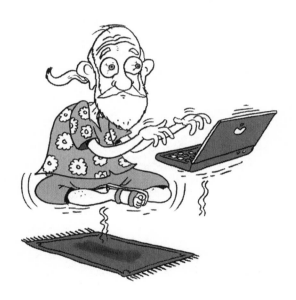

Dramatic Shift

Zen teaches that anyone who stops learning is old, whether at twenty or eighty...so true. For me, there has been a dramatic shift in thinking and looking at life. These experiences have helped me look deeper within, to assess what is really important and what isn't, to know myself better... to move from anguish to purpose.

I now feel there has been a remarkable improvement in how I view life. Since God's wake-up call fourteen months ago, every moment has been about the *present* and each day an opportunity to advance. I have begun experimenting with Eckhart Tolle's mental construct of the *now*, that: "Nothing exists outside this present moment" and have come to understand that if I am to experience anything positive in retirement, I must create it for myself in this moment. I'm doing things now from a state of joy instead of a feeling of obligation. I teach part time because I love teaching, not because I   need to earn money. I write because I enjoy writing and if at any moment I don't feel like writing, I don't write. Whenever I feel like taking several days off and fish or visit a place of interest, I do that. I am still not exactly at the place I want to be, but I'm sure as hell not where I was. Whoa! This is getting a little too weighty... let's move on.

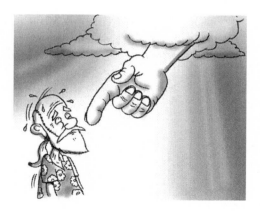

WHAT IS ZEN ANYWAY?

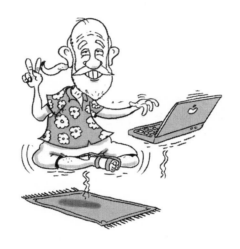

WHAT IS ZEN ANYWAY?

"The journey of one thousand miles begins with a flat tire."

Welcome to the Buddhahood. Pour yourself a tall, cool drink. What follows are the technical chapters. Every good book has some. Why would anyone write a book about Zen and retirement all in the same breath? And what's up with touting the merits of being a *frugalista* (new-age for cheapskate) in the process? Those are good questions. Let me put you at ease by saying upfront that this book is neither about "navel gazing" nor Buddhism (not even close). I'm not even an expert on Zen. I don't know anyone who truly is. For now, it is only important to know, as I have discovered, that these concepts all have symbiotic relationships. Let's give it a shot. I have written just enough about Zen to present you with a big picture of what I have learned Zen is or isn't. Anything more and you'll have to meditate on it yourself.

Every where you go, you hear Zen this and Zen that. So what is all this Zen stuff, anyway? Simply put, Zen is a sect of the Buddhist religion popularized in the sixties as a way of dealing with everyday challenges and annoyances of life. It is now being resurrected by baby boomers (who reigned in the height of the sixties) as a way of dealing with the frustrations of aging and retirement in an economy that's circling the toilet bowl and out-of-this-world technological advances.

Zen: It Is What It Is

First, let me put you at ease by saying that Zen isn't a distant or exotic concept. The peace and happiness you are seeking by applying Zen thinking to your everyday life is always right there in front of you, whether you're raking leaves or stuck in traffic. Second, when you begin to apply Zen thinking in retirement, you will find there are really no rules. Zen thinking doesn't involve any special knowledge or doctrine. It is not important to retreat to a mountain top or deep forest to meditate in the nude. You don't have to sit with your legs crossed to navel-gaze and make strange nasal sounds in order to understand the meaning of Zen. You don't even have to pray to any entity, shave your head or speak in a foreign tongue. You don't have to join a monastery, eat brown rice and yogurt or do Tai Chi in black pajamas looking like the guy in *The Matrix*. You don't even have to call it Zen. Zen just is.

Why Zen, Why Now?

Zen has now become a way of thinking and of being and plays an important part in today's aging and retirement. As you gradually apply a Zen attitude to your retirement, you will begin to develop new ways of thinking and of *being* in an imperfect world. You will no longer have to over-analyze, explain or justify anything to anyone. The world is not a perfect place and we have little control over what is going on. There is a rule of thumb I use when viewing the world. I like to say that the world runs on a *ninety-ten* rule: 90% great and 10% crappy. You're never going to get 100% satisfaction. If you can accept the notion that you're only going to get 90% of what you expect out of life that should be good enough. Then, in time, you'll get used to the 10% frustrations of life or find ways to make peace with them, and it'll be okay. Look, if everything were perfect and satisfactory, nothing would disappoint us. This would be heaven. We wouldn't need to seek spiritual fulfillment, enlightenment, or the ultimate truth. But since the world does suck a bit, 90% satisfaction should be good enough. That said, the application of Zen in retirement can help us place greater importance on letting go of petty annoyances and in making peace with the imperfect. And when we apply popular terms such as: *No big thing, whatever, it is what it is, fagetaboudit* and the popular *shit happens,* just know that we're not being passive-aggressive or dismissive, but that we are only reminding ourselves that the world is not a perfect place and that we need to stop demanding perfection of ourselves and others. That is Zen thinking... no more, no less.

No Time Like The Present

Zen also means living in the *now;* the present moment without the guilt-inducing chatter of our internal dialog. Zen teaches that with internal chatter comes confusion and if gone unchecked can be followed by exhaustion and depression, something you don't need at this stage of your life. That is why Zen is important. We are now at a juncture of our lives where we don't have time for any chaos and noise going on around (or within) us. The guilt-inducing shoulds and shouldn'ts, timelines, commitments and the general B.S. that guided our decisions before retirement should no longer matter. For us, there are now only two measurements of time: *Right now* and *the rest of my life.* How are you using your time? What do you want to do next? What are you willing to commit to until you draw your last breath and how will you do it? Michal Loewenthal, business trainer, illuminates this concept by saying that a belief in something is what gets us up in the morning and it's what often gets us through the toughest challenges. He points out that without something to believe in (crucial in retirement) we just wander around and hope that we find the door. This is also backed up by most (spiritually endowed) Zen Masters: "The great gate is always open, but people still look elsewhere."

Unloading Excess Baggage

In retirement, the application of Zen becomes one of waking up to the present moment and perceiving life and enjoying every aspect as it is going on around us rather than through the filtered lenses of our past experiences, prejudices and dualistic thinking (right vs. wrong; desirable vs. undesirable, good vs. bad). It can also be just carrying around some old guilt, failure or fear that impacted our previous relationships and

11

which made our life's journey difficult. This stuff is called "baggage" and can continue to negatively affect how we handle retirement.

I'm not all that great with analogies, but I have found them useful in explaining things that, at times, are difficult by relating them to something a person may already know. Retirement is like a journey; an adventure. But for this trip all you need is small carry-on luggage. All the excess baggage you've accumulated doesn't really matter anymore and is not needed. All excess baggage does is wear a person down and leads us to make comparisons, and as you may already be experiencing, comparisons lead to dissatisfaction, unnecessary guilt trips and stress that prevents us from enjoying our new adventure. The last thing we need at this stage of our lives is a bad trip.

I have come to several conclusions, but only one that I will share (at least for now). Retirement is a time to let go of all the old baggage (guilt, failed relationships, poor business decisions, obligations) and prioritize what goes into your carry-on bag. Good-bye tension...hello pension! The present trip is all there is! Prioritizing stuff is never easy, but once done it is well worth the pain and will make your journey so much more enjoyable. Get your needs met, once and for all! This is (literally) your final boarding call.

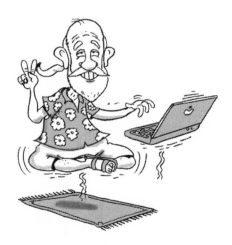

THE ZEN OF HUMOR

"Do we need to be foolish when funny?
Do we have to be serious when wise?
No!"

Zen teaches that life is funny and just as Zen accepts the world for what it is, a very illogical and funny place, we too must look at life and all it absurdities from a humorous point of view. In my walk through the wilderness I have learned that many things cannot be answered with logic. So I've tried to answer them with humor. Zen relies on humor to wrap a serious message in a humorous package, thus allowing us to experience certain truths. Zen breaks down the dualities between the sacred and the profane, meaning that with Zen, all great things are humbled and all "lowly" things are elevated onto a level playing field such as: "The truth will set you free, (the sacred) but first it will piss you off" (the profane). Conrad Hyers, in his *Zen and the Comic Spirit*, writes that Zen humor "...serves as a kind of comic midwife in the sense of a technique for precipitating (or provoking) an inner realization of the truth." This means that when Zen humor is broken down or has separated the sacred from the profane, it not only helps relieve tension, but often creates a greater awareness; a moving from "Ha ha!" to "Ah ha!" This becomes critical in retirement in that at last we can finally see the world for the illogical and funny place that it is and where we can now place greater value on the term "lighten up."

Enlighten Up!

Now laugh if you must, but smiling and laughter contain *Zen energy*. When we smile or laugh, our bodies release hormones and chemicals that have startling positive effects on our system. Laughter reduces stress, lowers blood pressure, lifts depression and adds years to your life. But you knew this already. What you didn't know is that many Eastern philosophers even go so far as to believe that the laughing *chakra* (a mystical-sounding Sanskrit term for "energy center"), shares or is very near the sex chakra. Just be careful you don't confuse the two or use them both at the same time with your soul mate or you'll be playing solitaire. And that would give out bad Karma (another cool Sanskrit term). Karma is a cosmic law that says if you do something *nice* to people, cool things will happen to you in return (either next week, next month, or in the next life). If you do something horrendous, well, you're screwed. (Does "what goes around, comes around" ring a bell?) I've read that because it's a cosmic law, you can't explain it nor can you get away from it. In fact, you may not fully understand it until you've crossed over into the next life, at which time you will have forgotten all about it and someday find yourself sitting alone with your face buried in your hands asking God, "Why me?" Now, that's Zen humor.

Zen And The Benefits Of Retirement

The benefits of Zen thinking in retirement are numerous. But, as I said, Zen is not Zen unless it is practiced. Then the benefits will manifest themselves. When you are finally able to meld Zen thought with aging and retirement, one benefit is that you no longer worry about the small stuff, because with Zen, everything is small stuff. I've listed below some undeniable benefits to aging and living a Zen retirement lifestyle:

1. There is nothing left to learn the hard way.

2. In a hostage situation, you're probably the first they'll release.

3. Your stories are looked upon as *oral history* and you can pontificate all you want.

4. You're the life of the party, but are forgiven for leaving at 10:00 pm.

5. Every day is casual Friday.

6. Lunchtime is when *you* decide.

7. There is only one law in the universe: NOW!

8. You never take your erections for granted. Ever.

9. If another person arrives at the potluck party with the same cheesy Hawaiian shirt and cutoffs, you might just become lifelong friends.

10. You can say "no" to people and feel okay about it.

11. You can finally balance your life.

12. You can Christmas shop for 15 relatives on December 23rd in sixty minutes.

13. You are a walking storeroom of trivia.

14. Your gray hair and crows feet add character.

15. You never have to hold your stomach in no matter who walks in the room.

16. Young women refer to you as "the cool older dude."

17. You can do your nails with a pocket knife.

18. You can adopt a sense of acceptance and humor in everything you see.

19. When gardening, the backyard is your urinal.

There you are. You don't have to thank me. Just remember that life's too short. Go ahead and break some rules. What could they possibly do to you? Throw off the shackles of other people's expectations and definition of propriety. Lots of mundane things are worthy of at least a chuckle. Now that you're retired (or soon be), start being yourself. Let people know the real you. They'll probably like you even better.

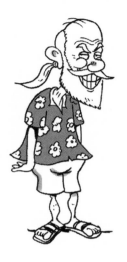

FEARS, DOUBTS, AND OTHER BUMMERS

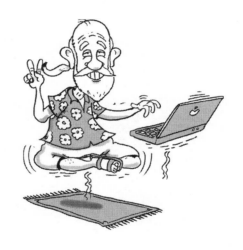

FEARS, DOUBTS AND OTHER BUMMERS

"If you understand, things are just as they are.
If you don't understand, things are just as they are."

I've made a few other observations during my time spent figuring out this retirement stuff: 1) Age happens and it's out of my control and 2) Retirement has a very short pleasure curve if all I'm going to do is sit around. For some, perpetual idleness can be a real bummer. It is little wonder that most men are easily (and needlessly) bummed out three months after retirement happens. There's the worry of the obvious (the nest egg issue). But deeper within lies the mother of all bummers, what Elisabeth Coleman, speaker and author refers to as "Post-Institutional Stress Syndrome" (PISS), a psychological condition that is associated with having to transition from a career to retirement.

Mother Of All Bummers

PISS: Here's how it works. You first begin to experience some depression, restlessness and some really screwed up sleeping patterns, only to wake up tired and exhausted. Up until retirement, you had been that type "A" guy who used to wake up at dawn and begin cranking out e-mails. You were the first one at the office with one-third of the day's work done. You might even say that the minute your feet would hit the bedroom floor in the morning, even Satan would shudder, "Shit! He's awake."

Things seem different now. You still get up to shower and shave. "Why?" you wonder. You aren't going anywhere. You begin to dress sloppier than before. And why not, you don't have any meetings on your schedule. (You don't even have a schedule!) You've been retired three months and you've already painted every room in the house (Twice!). You find yourself rearranging lawn furniture, moving plants and killing wasps until five o'clock when the senior citizen dinner specials begin. After dinner, you go home and sip wine through the six o'clock news and fall asleep during a nine o'clock reality show. You suddenly find that "Mr. Happy" (figure it out) is no longer responding like before you retired, except when you have to pee and that's every three hours. While your mind used to be able to retain and access data like a computer, it now crashes and burns and concentration problems begin to interfere with your personal and social life. You've hit a wall. Those are all PISS symptoms (Okay, risk factors) that threaten good mental and physical health. There's more. Read on.

Shoulda, Woulda, Coulda

Nothing prepared me for the changes I went through the first six months of retirement. It was a time when all the retirement fears came crawling out of the woodwork. There was the destructive self-doubt baggage (shoulda, woulda, coulda) and the dreaded "F" word: *FEAR*... Fear of aging, fear of loneliness, fear of being a burden, fear of poverty and the big one, fear of dying. Though most men can overcome these obstacles, many go undiagnosed and remain spiritually paralyzed by it, resulting in physical and mental issues. Maybe this is you at this moment and how you wound up at this section of the bookstore.

You begin to feel lonely and isolated. Within a few months, you begin to long for the time when you were a *somebody* with a title and a reputation, where others (identity managers) were taking good care of what Eckhart Tolle calls your "external identity"...defining yourself by your professional position or title. Now retirement has you confused. You shudder at the thought of losing that identity and dealing with the sudden (and irrational) fear of becoming invisible, a nobody…not even owning a business card. You look in the mirror and you don't even know who the hell you are, what makes you unique, what you value and who you are in terms of your personality, character and principles. You don't know what to say about yourself when meeting strangers so you make up stories like: "I'm home officing. Uh, I'm exploring other options." Or the biggest lie of all, "I'm a freelance consultant." Riiight!

You've suddenly begun to realize that after it's all said and done, material things and external relationships come and go, but in the final analysis, who you are, is ultimately what you really get to keep. Am I bumming you out? Sorry. But those are all risk factors that compromise mental, physical and emotional health. If you're experiencing these, get thee to a doctor or seek other professional help ASAP. In time, change will come, but only if you let it.

Enough Already!

I soon realized that I was slowly being sucked in by a pool of quicksand; that "spiritual death" when gone unchecked, can often lead to self-doubt, depression, and alcohol or prescription drug abuse. It took six months to claw my way out of this pool of self-pity. Being an old street fighter (and with a little counseling help), I screamed, "Enough already!"

By now you may have gathered that I was a Psych major in college. Don't panic. I'm not going to burden you with a lot of recycled, new-age jargon, but here's what I think. All these fears are nothing more than products of irrational and self-defeating thinking. For example, fear of being overwhelmed by life's challenges at this stage of your life can lead to health and mental issues which in turn can transform you into that grumpy old S.O.B. I talked about in the introduction, something you don't want to be. I have begun to learn that for one to become a freer, more confident retiree, one must sort out all this stuff and break through those fears that have prevented us from moving forward. Sometimes we have to stop listening to all our internal "buts", "what-ifs", and excuses.

Freedom (liberation to be more exact), is about the ability to fear less and do more and can only be accomplished through a process of introspection, acceptance (it is what it is), and making that decision to just let stuff go. At this stage of our lives, the present moment is all we ever have and maintaining the quality of it should be our only primary focus. If you cannot find freedom right where you are, then where do you expect to find it.

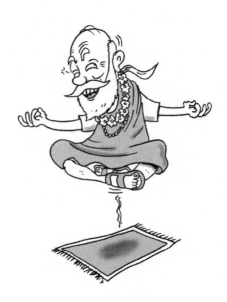

REALITY CHECK

"Things are not what they seem; nor are they otherwise."

It's funny how everyone wants to live a long time, but no one wants to grow old. In fact, we seem to fear aging more than our own mortality. The other day, while ordering at a 1950s throwback restaurant, I found myself looking at the senior's menu and realizing I was old enough to order from it. But I'm not going to do that, EVER! Am I in denial? Perhaps.

For some of us, retirement heightens our awareness of aging. Some of us go so far as to say that getting old is like eating at an all-you-can-eat buffet: What should be hot is cold. What should be hard is limp. And what looks enticing, we can no longer touch. So we pass it up. And it doesn't really matter because there are some men who have discovered that they can now go for weeks without sex, but not one day without their glasses. (It's been so long since I've had sex I've forgotten who ties up whom.) Your first impulse when encountering this dilemma might be to do what many men do, that is read up on foolish methods to keep young... from liposuction around your love handles to wonder drugs to keep you going.

And why not? It works on laboratory monkeys. Oh, yeah, and don't forget increasing your credit card limit. After all, you're only as young as your credit card let's you be, right? Wrong. In a short time you'll find that you've been electronically transferring money (for some young hottie) faster than Paul McCartney did during his divorce negotiations. All that stuff you've been reading about, wonder drugs and living la vida loca is a lot of hype. Sorry, but there are no shortcuts to keeping young. So much for growing old gracefully.

Aging need not be the big bad bummer some people make it out to be. It can be a very healthy and rewarding way to spend the better third of your life, provided you exercise and stay active. Research has shown that staying active, especially at something you love, reverses the aging process. I don't have the data to support this, but it's a safe bet that when you become productive and live with a purpose you'll notice that you begin to feel healthier, walk a little crisper and look a little younger...almost to the point that you begin to lie a little about your age. Knocking off three to five years is not bad for anyone. Any more than that and you're a raving liar. But why lie in the first place? If you've got it, flaunt it! Still, there are some men stuck in denial who are too lazy to explore more practical and healthier options to aging.

Denial Ain't Just A River In Egypt

Of all things, aging is the most unexpected thing that happens to men. Second is being accidentally shot in the face in a hunting accident by Dick Cheney. See if I'm way out in left field on this one. One morning you wake up and look in the mirror and say, "Damn! This can't be me." All this time you were thinking that everybody else was aging except you. You've been in denial... generally a man's first survival instinct. "No way," you say. Look, I've been around the block enough times to know that when someone is denying they are in denial, they are only proving they are really in denial. Just man-up to it and own it.

The denial phase is generally followed by the desire to recover lost ground...to look young once again. You now think you have to spend hard-earned money for a membership in a high class fitness club then rush out to buy the latest men's hair coloring kit and a jar of industrial strength Viagra. And why not? It's the easiest (and most expedient) thing to do. It has now become necessary for your self-esteem, to look and dress young, yet each time you pass the mirror you become more disappointed at what you see. You then enroll in a hormone replacement therapy program just to improve your quality of life (code for getting laid more). You begin dressing like a young John Travolta and drinking high-end energy drinks. And for what? It doesn't change the equation... and it could kill you.

Let's get real here. Just man-up to the fact that you've aged a bit and that it's okay. Stop pretending that you're a twenty-something strutting your stuff around the mall in your vintage "Members Only" jacket and that silly "I refuse to age" baseball cap (with the tune *Duke of Earl* humming in your head). Don't look now, but your stuff has strutted off without you. I think we look older (and more ridiculous) when we try to dress to look like we're competing with a disco Dan or some aging rocker. Don't think that by dyeing your hair and spending good money on the latest pair of tennis shoes, designer jeans and that fear-of-mortality earring you got at the mall will make you a chick magnet. Here's what I think. As you get older, the pickings get slimmer (but your waist doesn't). Odds are, dressed like that, the best you're going to do is attract a fifty-plus, overly made-up babe in inappropriately tight leather pants whose stomach is making the same gurgling noises as her coffee maker and who can't wait to get home to get in her jammies.

But on the other hand, there are some pretty attractive over-fifty women that still turn heads. The unfortunate part is that for every stunning, fifty-plus lady out there, there are ten paunchy dudes in gold chains and designer jeans making fools of themselves in front of twenty year old waitresses.

Through The Looking Glass

Look, we all have a distorted view of ourselves. Not to depress you, but just look in the mirror. You don't look like a young John Travolta. C'mon, you look like your father. Are you still with me? Have I been a little too blunt? All I'm saying is that be careful with   the denial aspect of aging, as it eventually leads to anger, depression and distress then one day, surprise! You'll discover that you've become incapacitated and your children are drawing straws to see whose turn it will be to sit with you in the senior assisted living home on Sunday afternoon.

Retirement need not be the big fat downer people make it out to be. Just be proud and enjoy where you are at this moment in time. Buy a used Corvette if you feel the need. That's cool. Buy a vintage Harley and date a young woman if you can afford the high maintenance. What makes people assume only teenagers have a monopoly on being outrageous or rebellious? You can still do it, but do it in a mature way.

You don't have to dress and look like an old fogey. That's insane. Just dress like a youngish, but cool adult. I refuse to believe that as a man matures he becomes increasingly uncool. Life doesn't end at sixty, nor does class and style. The point here is that fantasies can be fun, but self-delusion isn't flattering to anyone.

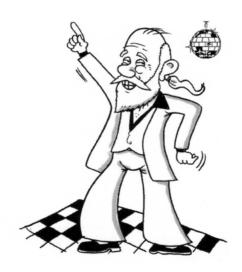

DEATH-PROOFING
YOUR LIFE

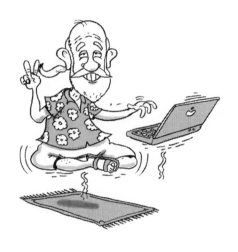

DEATH-PROOFING YOUR LIFE

"Knowledge is learning something every day.
Wisdom is letting go of something every day."

I remember back in the day when my mother would take out the quilts on the first week of spring and give them a good shaking to remove all the crud that had accumulated all winter, then hang them on the line for a couple of days. She instinctively knew it was time for a clean "change." We knew that we had entered a new season and soon we would be out outside playing ball just a little later, knowing that that evening, instead of heavy quilts, we would be sleeping under clean, fresh sheets. There was a sense of exhilaration attached to this seasonal ritual. In a sense, we felt free!

Now that seems a little wacky for some guys, but retirement is like that. It is a time when we can give our minds a good shaking and finally remove all the layers of accrued opinions, beliefs, prejudices, frozen expectations and the B.S. that stood between us and true freedom. And this is also when the greater challenge begins: acquiring true freedom.

It's funny how we can value freedom so much, but often cannot achieve it until we have no other choice. The application of Zen thinking in retirement does this. You will learn, as I did, that freedom (true freedom) is a greater challenge than power...that thing we had to maintain back

29

at the cubicle village we had been chained to all those years. Think about it. Back then, you were all about being Mr. Big and all about what (and whom) you could control. You were defined by *what* you were and what you did, not by *who* you were as a person. To use me as an example, I went so far as to purchase a black-on-black, fully loaded, gas-guzzling SUV with a personalized license plate that screamed: "Dr. Lou!" I wasn't even that kind of a doctor. If someone fainted in a theatre and the management announced, "Is there a doctor in the house?" I wasn't the guy you wanted. For me, life was all about maintaining my *external* identity. As I previously stated, external identity is nothing more than defining ourselves as being something we're not and wanting others to recognize us as unique. This helps enlarge our self-worth through an endless list of external identifiers such as the Armani suits we wear, that huge SUV we drive, the wines we drink, and the office we work in (corner-glass vs. gray-cubicle). The list is endless. What I really lacked was a strong *internal* identity…that sense of who I really am.

What Does Death-Proofing Mean Anyway?

Death-proofing? Sounds spooky. Death-proofing is nothing more than a term used by new-age folks to identify and implement preventive measures that prolong youth and extend life. It could be diet, exercise, fun and productive activities or just having a positive mental attitude about stuff. The Dalai Lama, the religious leader of Tibet (and a large following of stringy-haired backpackers), refers to it as letting go of negative thoughts and destructive habits and replacing them with opposing positive ones that are stronger and more powerful. Recovery folks call it *self-care*. No matter what your philosophy, it's still death-proofing your life.

The Zen Of Letting Go

Zen teaches that giving up or walking away from a situation doesn't always mean we are weak. Sometimes it means that we are strong enough to set a boundary, to say no, to change an old pattern, or just to let go of persons or things that have caused us anxiety in the past. Retirement is a good time to get a sense of knowing who we are, what we value then looking at the chaos around us and asking ourselves, "Is this that important?" and then letting it go.

It is time to make that change and you know it. You may find yourself under attack at first from those who are used to the old you and don't want you to change. That's okay. It is not your fault that people can't handle your newfound freedom. You're now looking out for number ONE and have the right to take care of yourself. Don't let other people's reactions guilt you into submission. Just stay the course.

Retirement is also a time to tap into our inner boundlessness and explore doing greater things for ourselves and others. Dean Sluyter, author of *Zen Commandments,* points to freedom as no longer being about what or whom we can control or the power plays we can freely make, but more about focusing on how much of our potential we can now unleash. That is also a part of death-proofing your life…doing things that matter and which result in a longer and more productive life.

The challenge lies in our inability as men to stand back and take a long, hard look at ourselves and determine just what the hell we came on this earth to accomplish. Dean Sluyter describes it as looking deeper within ourselves and taking better inventory of our talents and gifts and then laying a solid foundation for what we want the rest of our lives to look like. For some of us, that can be some pretty scary stuff. We've never been challenged to look within and make that deep of an assessment.

Laying A Solid Foundation

Death-proofing one's life takes time and a little hard work. It's like building any new project; a patio for example. Some groundwork has to be laid. You have to first dig out all the decayed roots and branches that have accumulated underground over the years. You can't just bury all that stuff, smooth out the dirt, hide everything under fresh concrete and expect to have a lasting patio. The same is true when death-proofing your life. Burying all past experiences, prejudices, and bad habits as if they never happened may look good on the surface, but the old, weak and decayed foundation won't sustain the new fresh one you're trying to create and in a short time (like the patio), it will collapse. Soon you'll be back nursing those fears and self-doubts.

Strategies For Death-Proofing Your Life

It is never too late to begin death-proofing your life. Looking back, I think of the lyrics to the song "My Way" (Frank's version, of course): *Regrets, I've had a few, but then again too few to mention.* Okay, I'll mention one or two. First, I never got rich, really rich. Every time I got close, someone raised the bar. So, I've kept myself busy all my adult life tilting at windmills in the world of non-profits. Second, I also never learned how to body surf well. My son from California says I surf like a garden boulder. Remember when learning how to play Led Zeppelin's *Stairway to Heaven* on a guitar was the coolest thing ever? I never learned that one either. What does all this regression have to do with death-proofing your life? Plenty. It's never too late to revisit priorities and learn new stuff (except maybe body surfing). There are many things you can do to begin building a foundation for death-proofing your life. Pick the one you like and do it!

1. Get out from behind the TV or computer screen. Don't neglect your real-world relationships in favor of virtual interaction.

2. Be with people who nurture your needs. Choose friends, neighbors, colleagues, and family members who are upbeat, positive, and interested in you.

3. Take care of your body; exercise; rest.

4. Make leisure time a priority.

5. Do the things that turn you on. (Beyond sex. But do that also. It's one of the all time greats.)

6. Stop eating crap. Crap affects your energy and mood.

7. Learn to say, "No!" Without this skill you will be too overloaded with other people's priorities instead of your own.

8. Schedule an event (sporting event, museum, etc.) once a week and stick to it.

9. Become an adjunct teacher at a community college or adult education program. English-as-a-second language is always a fun thing to teach.

10. Start a new hobby.

11. Learn to cook...lose yourself in the kitchen.

12. Sip a little wine after a hard day's work in the garden...survey your kingdom. Take it all in.

13. Pray, meditate, start a journal.

14. Join a club.

15. Record your family history...a visit to your country of origin is of great historical importance and fun.

16. Learn to play an instrument. It's not too late to play *Stairway to Heaven* on a guitar.

17. Take a chef's course in your town or a foreign country (only if it fits your budget).

18. Become a teacher's aide in a low-income community elementary school.

19. Get a pilot's license (if flying is your thing).

20. Hold a garage sale once a month. Use the rest of the month to visit other garage sales, meet new people, buy their junk, and sell it at yours.

21. Plant a garden.

22. Take a horticulture class at your local college.

23. Join a writing club.

24. Download music and give CDs to your friends.

25. Start a vintage vinyl records collection.

26. Study new religions.

27. Throw a monthly movie/dinner party with a group of close friends by going to a matinee (it's cheaper between 12:00 and 4:00 p.m.) then discuss it as a group over a potluck dinner at home.

28. Learn a foreign language.

29. Become a mystery shopper. It pays $100 per day.

30. Do something unpredictable (like yoga).

31. Start your own personal web page/blog and pontificate for awhile.

32. Evaluate your commitments. Think about which ones you really give a damn about and which ones you can toss without incurring guilt or stress.

33. Live with passion and purpose.

Just keep in mind that everyone is different, with different situations, stages, emotions and so on. Not all things will be equally beneficial to all people. Not all of the suggestions I've listed will work for you. Still, select one or two and try them out. Take it slow, experiment. Find activities that you enjoy and that give you a mental and physical boost. Then throw yourself into them. Ride them out for all they're worth.

You'll soon see the difference it makes in your life. I don't know how else to convince you. You may just have to discover it yourself. Zen Masters teach that in order to make sense out of change, one must plunge into it, move with it, and join the dance.

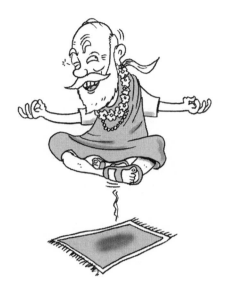

THE "WE" GENERATION

Lucky me! Being of a generation that doesn't easily accept defeat, it only took one year to adapt to my new lifestyle. But not without a little pain. This retirement thing is not for the faint of heart. But it's nothing to worry about either. After all, have you forgotten who we are? Wake up! We're Baby Boomers... newly retired members of the *WE* generation that now makes up 25% of the population and own 77% of the world's financial assets.

WE have raised more than our fair share of hell during the half-century we've been on the planet. *WE* created dialogue...much of it shouted. If we didn't get our political way we threw public tantrums (demonstrations). *WE*'ve always rebelled against tradition and made up our own rules. For example: *WE* fought injustices and an unpopular war. *We* created rock and roll, Woodstock, the word "groovy" and (for good or bad) disco. *WE* invented the computer, the cell phone and Viagra. *WE* were the first social activists and the first to give the system the finger and fight for (and change attitudes toward) women and gay rights. And, *WE* are the generation that began the Civil Rights Movement that 44 years later elected the first African-American President. But it doesn't end there.

Here we are today, brighter, more experienced, richer, experiencing an unprecedented amount of leisure and once again taking on *Big Brother* only this time by redefining retirement and old age. Be afraid. Be very afraid. We know how to walk the talk. We're not ready to raise the white flag.

Sixty: The New Forty (You Say?)

The Golden Years? Are you kidding me? Sounds terminal. I'm a sixty-something (67 ½ to be precise) and still navigating a brand-new path... and having the time of my life. I've taken up art photography, writing, teaching and will soon learn Italian in preparation for my first European trip...and all at my own pace. To quote an old television commercial from back in the day, "You're not getting older; you're getting better." (But only if you exercise.) People like to toss Hugh Hefner's quote around, "Eighty is the new forty." That's fine if you can afford weekly testosterone therapy and seaweed smoothies.

Sixty as the new forty sounds more realistic. It's prime time. We've barely put our toes into the new millennium. We're at the top of our game now and there are a lot of things left to learn and do and they're happening at the speed of light. Just because we've retired doesn't mean we've become incompetent or obsolete...a relic. The jugular question now becomes, what are we going to do with the remaining twenty or thirty years?

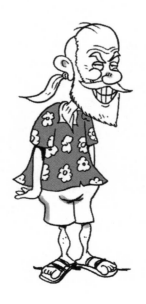

LIVING WITH PURPOSE

**"People love others not for who they are but for how
they make them feel"**

One good way I found to death-proof my life was to keep feeling useful,
tapping into my past skills (stuff I already knew) and applying them to
my retirement. I began to turn my pre-retirement experiences and skills
into post-retirement tools. The knowledge and skills I had accumulated
all these years as a grant writer, teacher, counselor and administrator,
both in the private and public sectors had provided me with a toolbox
full of creative skills that could be used to help others. These skills
opened the doors for substitute teaching, counseling, grant writing and
business planning for newly developed charter schools and other new
start-up youth-serving agencies. You can do the same!

Let's say that you were once a high-end CPA for some large firm. Doesn't
it seem natural to use those skills and experiences to begin doing some
good? Pro bono accounting work, for example, for a small, struggling
non-profit comes to mind, or tax work in low-income communities,
or math tutoring in a small urban school. I could go on. The point is
the peace and the spiritual rewards you seek will return to you tenfold.
Bill Gates nails it when he says, "Until we're educating every kid in a
fantastic way, until every inner city is cleaned up, there is no shortage
of things to do."

Sweet Mellissa

I recently volunteered at a school/facility for kids with special needs and was assigned to a group of pretty amazing 12-15 year olds. Music, as you would guess, played an important role in their therapy. I noticed that Mellissa, a quadriplegic, would be pushed to a corner of the room by an aide because, according to the aide, Mellissa was too shy to participate in a crowd and, could only vocalize with grunts and screeches and could only move one hand at the wrist. Because her neck was also weak, the most she could do was stare at the floor as the Disney songs played. (Why Disney, when, regardless of their handicapping conditions, these kids were teens?!!) After a week of this, I got tired of playing *Little Mermaid* stuff and became bold enough to go to my car during a brief break and come back with my *Queen's Greatest Hits* CD to play in the classroom. I announced to the class that everyone had to dance or sing for a prize. As the class went wild jumping and making their best attempts to maintain a beat to *We will, we will rock you*, Mellissa slowly raised her head, made a fist and vigorously began shaking it up and down and sideways to the beat of the music. Wow!

That month I left for other school sites and in about three weeks returned to the school for another assignment. I spied Mellissa slumped in her wheelchair in the hallway with her aide at her side. Not knowing if she remembered me, I called out her name in my familiar friendly growl: Mellissaahh! And, as she slowly raised her head to see who was calling her name, she caught my presence and her eyes immediately lit up. In what seemed like a longer gaze than normal, I could see a real person deep in those eyes; a person with feelings and personal history. Apparently remembering the class exercise we had done repeatedly, she knowingly began shaking her fist up and down and sideways to some dance rhythm in her head. In my thirty years in education, that has been my most moving moment.

Recently a cousin and good friend Phil sent me a copy of Rick Warren's *Purpose Driven Life* and I actually read it. Phil's gift brought me to the realization that we all have a purpose in life... that God doesn't play dice with the universe. We were not put on this earth by some random accident or be a background character in someone else's movie. You might say that we all came here on purpose. My purpose was not necessarily higher education or being a mover and shaker. It was in leaving kids (some of which have never had their spirit touched) just a little happier than when I first met them and for me to grow from that experience.

What's It All About?

What is our destiny? How do we want to be remembered? Do our lives have a purpose beyond the daily grind or material success?

How do we find what that is? What's it all about? These are the questions that have eluded us through the ages. Not to sound overly therapeutic, but let me just say that we all are put on this earth for a specific purpose. Without purpose, life lacks meaning and offers little fulfillment. No wonder we ask these questions. They are central to a happy and productive life. A "Life Review Survey" of older Americans conducted by the University of California in 1993 showed that one of the best predictors of life satisfaction and happiness is whether a person considers his or her life to have purpose (interestingly, not income). Happy and unhappy people are not born that way. Both types do things that create or reinforce their moods. Happy people live life with a purpose and do things that allow themselves to be happy. Happy people have a strategy (a plan) for maintaining happiness and then go about making it happen. It's that simple. Unhappy people, on the other hand, continue doing things that upset them and which reinforces their unhappiness. Wayne Dyer talks about this topic with ease. He says that there is only one cause of unhappiness: the false beliefs you have in your head, beliefs so widespread, so commonly held, that it never occurs to you to question them. I'm no Wayne Dyer, but I believe that happiness is knowing the source of our unhappiness, and then doing something to finally change it.

How are you using your time? Feeling frustrated? Now don't get overwhelmed. Finding your purpose in life is not an immediate must-do thing. Nor is it about doing, but more about *being* and taking the time to discover it. It might be lodged very deep within, but it's there nonetheless. In time, it will soon become apparent or, like me, you'll stumble upon it. But until you do, begin living life to the fullest and in the present. You've held yourself back too long. (Others may have held you back too long.) Let yourself try something new. Maybe you'll like it. Maybe you won't…and does it matter?

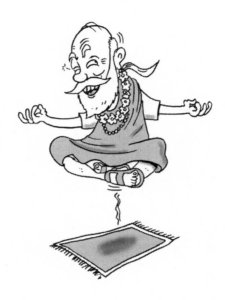

ZEN AND THE ART OF
RATIONAL SELF-INTEREST

"We are in absolute charge of ourselves."

Meditate on this. "Rational self-interest" has now become the new *selfish*. Retirement is going to be a time to meet your own needs, letting materialistic things and troublesome people go. It's going to mean getting selfish. Selfish is a word that has taken a bad rap over the years. But selfish is nothing more than a Zen concept for self-advocacy and letting go of things that cause you discomfort or pain. New age Zen Masters call it *rational self interest*. It means nurturing your *self*, by doing those things that make you feel safe, good or complete without feeling guilty. The problem, writes Melody Beattie in her *The Language of Letting Go,* is that we end up apologizing every time we try to stick up for ourselves…that guilt can prevent us from setting boundaries that are often in our best interest. It makes sense, especially in retirement. You are free now and should not be allowed to be controlled by guilt. You're going to have to act as if what you are doing for yourself makes all the difference in the world. And it does. Now the fun begins.

The Darker Side Of Zen

Welcome to the dark side. Staying young, vibrant and independent is finally within your control. Suddenly, you notice people at the mall pausing to look at you. You've got this proud (but not arrogant) look about you that you've never had before. You walk among the masses in daily life, but you're not a part of them. You've got this feeling of earned superiority...you've found yourself and it's about time. You're your own man! My kids call it *swagger*...retirement swagger. I just call it freedom. No, liberation...my personal transformation.

So what if some people can't handle your swagger? You can now say what you want, be a tad provocative and raise some eyebrows from time to time. You can be noticed, admired, disliked or loved.
These are good things because, at the very least, people will find you interesting. It's about being different from the masses, but being honest. But not so honest that your spouse has to step on your air hose every time you open your mouth. Don't go over the top. Never make fun of people's God, their sexuality, their politics or anything they hold dear. There is nothing wrong with taking a surprising (but harmless) position or making an outlandish (but intelligent) analogy and all the time with your tongue pressed firmly in your cheek. You've now got retirement swagger. Just use it wisely.

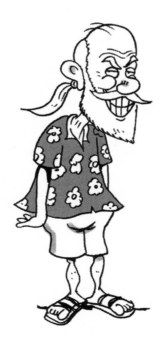

STAY BUSY, DO LESS

"When you're over the hill you pick up speed."

I admire Anton Chekhof the Russian writer who, while dying of tuberculosis, was still able to complete building a house. You don't believe it? Google it.

I can hear your pain already, "What if I get bored after a few months of doing nothing? What if I still want to work? My wife doesn't want me around the house messing up her established routine. Who will I socialize with?" These are all legitimate questions. As I have already stated, the first year after retirement can be full of emotions. You might experience a combination of relief, anxiety, excitement, and confusion about your new identity (or non-identity). You miss being in the eye of the storm, solving problems and being bothered by idiots. I understand. You've suddenly learned that, for you, the pleasure curve of retirement is short and are feeling totally bummed out at being disconnected and out of the loop. You're running out of things to do and your spouse is threatening to relocate you to a condo in Florida (Medicare by the sea). And last year she had you on a cruise to Alaska where you sadly saw the same icebergs going up as coming back, say nothing of spending five days tethered to your spouse in a rigged casino, feeding a slot machine and eating foods that were too exotic for your system, all in the name of bonding. There may be some romance in growing old together, but then there's the reality. To steal Tony Soprano's Zen quote, "Fagetaboudit!"

By now, you're beginning to feel that maybe all those great death-proofing tips I've just listed may not be for you. Relax. These feelings are entirely normal. However, if you still haven't risen above the funk you're in, then maybe a job, a place where you feel you are needed and appreciated may be the answer. It's really okay. For some people, to paraphrase a line from Bob Critchley's book *Rewire or Rust*, "It is better to wear out than rust out," meaning that since we're living longer, just focusing on the leisure side of retirement may not be enough. We must revisit our new "life roles" and modify them to maintain a more fulfilling life. His book supports the assertion that some people get greater emotional and physical perks from working (until they fall over and are quietly hauled away) than sitting around in perpetual idleness. To some, work and being around people provides identity, status, income and a host of other things. It connects us to people. Not working causes us to lose much of our meaning and identity. The trick now is to stay busy, but do less. Let me show you how it works.

The Zen Of Re-Wiring

It's no secret that the workplace and the concept of work have changed. New technology, an aging population and a looming skills shortage are having a monumental effect on the way we work today and how we will work in the future. These days, many people work from home and are connected through phones, the Internet and other gadgets to the degree that the concept of *work* has now become ambiguous and more difficult to define.

The definition of a working retiree has also been redefined. So much so that no one is exactly sure what it means. "What does that have to do with me?" you ask. Plenty. Write these stats along the margin: According to a 2004 study by the U.S. Bureau of Labor Statistic, 25% of people age 65 to 74 are now in the workforce and the reason for working is not necessarily for income. In 2005, 24% of the workforce age 62 to 64 was self-employed.

Most people are now viewing post-retirement careers for enjoyment, curiosity and for the challenge, even if they are already well set financially. And what's wrong with bringing in a few extra bucks? Research shows that retired people who work, especially those in jobs they enjoy, tend to be happier and live longer than those who don't. Working retirees are now doing less and because of their vast experience are focusing only on the important things...delegating the rest.

Maybe that's what you need to do. I recommend, however, that you try and get the best of both worlds by convincing your boss or board of directors to sub-contract with you on a part time basis so you can serve both as trainer and mentor to the young Turks that are clawing their way up the corporate ladder. If you performed well over the years, they'll let you do it and give you a fat bonus to boot. Now you don't have to sweat age discrimination issues if that has even been a concern. You're a reliable known product. It's the perfect win-win plan.

What About Age Discrimination?

What about it? Look, if you're going to be looking for full time work, perhaps age discrimination will be a factor. However, as a retiree, you are looking to feel productive and take command of yourself. Working part time does this.

As a retiree looking for work, you face great advantages. You've got experience. You're flexible and knowledgeable. You're no longer a lean-and-mean hungry go-getter. You're comfortable in your own skin. You're an elder and a mentor. You command respect. Just get out and sell yourself and your experiences and don't let fears about age discrimination stop you. Hell, age and experience are assets...not deficits. Don't forget the Lee Iacocca story about age and experience: A young bull and an old bull stood on a hill surveying a herd of cows. The young bull, eager to mate, broke out in a sweat and stomping and snorting said, "Pops, let's *run* down there and get us one!" The old bull calmly replied, "Slow down, son. Let's *walk* down there and get them all." Now that's experience.

Look Up-To-Date

Ditch the wide tie and white belt. Look up-to-date. Your dress must reflect today's attire and will add the credibility you will need around a young workforce. You may be working for a guy in his twenties. Don't risk looking like an artifact. You have a lot to offer and if you look like some old fogey from the past, you may be portrayed as someone who doesn't have current up-to-date work skills.

Bottom line: You've got to be flexible and resourceful, maybe even more than when you were climbing your career ladder. Whether you're contemplating getting out in the workforce on your own terms or not, always look marketable. Polish up your resume, become technology literate, and prepare to network (at your age, passive job hunting on the internet may not be enough). Mary Lloyd, author of *Super-Charged Retirement,* calls networking "The other web." She points to the importance of having a network (connections) of contacts you can tap into as you make that critical transition to what you want to do next in life. The problem we face when retiring, she cautions, is that most of us feel we will no longer need to access our business contacts and we let those connections atrophy. Big mistake. Too, visibility outside your business network is just as important in retirement. Meeting with active retirees who may have the same interests as you can be healthy and fun. You may not want to work anymore, but you may still want to become a part of a group that may need reliable person with your skills to help you see a community project through. Leave all doors open.

LIVING LA VIDA CHEAP!

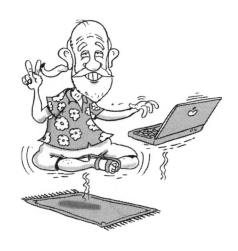

LIVING LA VIDA CHEAP

"Give a man a fish and he will eat for a day. Teach a man to fish and he will sit in his boat all day drinking beer."

The good old days are gone and they aren't ever coming back: Failed banks, panicked markets, rising unemployment social security is taking a dive and our nest egg continues to shrink. We're in a world of shit. Desperate times call for desperate measures. One purpose for writing this book was to reach out to as many retirees during these turbulent economic times as I could and provide them with some practical ideas on living a frugal, yet happy lifestyle. I believe in being proactive and there's no time like the present to assess our current retirement situation and prepare for the long, drawn out recession ahead.

Untroubled Retirement In Troubled Times

Life is short and I believe in the importance of not living beyond my means. Take it from one who knows, there's a great deal of comfort and satisfaction to be had in having a little money stashed away so that we're not devastated by the next crisis. I can hear your next question, "But does it mean that by being a frugalista I'll be living a Spartan existence searching under sofa cushions for change just to eat out?" No, not really. Like Robert Kiyosaki's book *Rich Dad, Poor Dad* suggests: wait, save, find the deals and when you have the cash, go for it. That is the life of a true frugalista. Kiyosaki suggests that a frugalista makes compromises and tries to strike a balance while remaining financially secure. Makes sense. Details to follow. For now, let's just look at the big picture.

Frugal: The New Cheap

I know, I know. Your first response is to become turned off by the word *cheap* and *cheapskate* and why not? In this shop-till-you-drop society, being cheap is made fun of and we've been trained since birth to believe that a cheapskate is a guy with short arms and tight pockets. In today's economy, all that has changed. This is the point where I opt for a "lifeline" and use Webster's Dictionary as my resource.

There are many meanings for cheap that range from "a bargain" to "of comparatively small value." You might say that *cheap* has gotten a bad rap. But if you look deeper, the meaning expands to a more positive definition like "low in price or cost...not expensive, a great deal, costing little labor or trouble and a favorable bargain." Now when you shop for cool bargains, you're not cheap anymore...you're frugal. Frugal and cheap are now interchangeable terms. Don't believe it? Why, then, are there businesses sprouting up with titles like: Cheap Flights, Cheapo Records, Cheap Rentals, Cheap Web Hosting, Dollar Daze, and the Dollar Store which has grown into a billion dollar business and continues to pride itself on, and proudly market frugal as the way to save money? Welcome, frugalistas!

Frugalista: The New Cheapskate

For starters, living frugally is probably one of the most misunderstood concepts. One of my biggest pet peeves about the words frugal and cheap is that they imply that retirees are a bunch of penny-pinching, crabby, old bastards. Obviously, this is a major misconception of the outside world.

Maybe I'm wrong, but let me say this in our defense. We are happy, but scrappy fighters who eat well, enjoy the quality and value of the items we purchase and happen to enjoy stashing away any savings for extra fun stuff. We pinch dollars, not pennies! What is wrong with that? With the cash we stash, we can do whatever we want, whenever we want, as much as we want and we have more fun doing it. Maybe that's what those on the outside don't like. And do we care?

Living as a frugalista is nothing more than knowing how to efficiently use our money to better meet our retirement needs. It doesn't really require missing out on the pleasures of life. In fact, the opposite is true. A frugal lifestyle allows us to simplify our lives because we're spending less. Zen teaches that the less stuff we have, the less stressful our lives become. It makes good practical sense.

The less we spend, the less we need to earn, resulting in stashing more cash and spending more time at what we love. And who doesn't want that? In the end, nothing in life is permanent anyway and all the stuff you've hoarded is just that...stuff! Never confuse stuff for success.

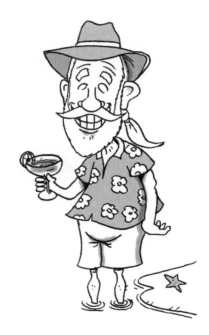

TOUGH TIMES CALL FOR DRASTIC MEASURES

"Nothing happens next. This is it."

Living on a limited budget and facing what the government has done with our economy, there are days when I can't even tell if I'm on Golden Pond (the Fonda movie) or up the creek.

Tough economic times call for drastic measures. I have learned through having to make my own personal retirement adjustments and through conversations with other retired men in my situation that we all wish we could stretch our small nest egg, but many of us don't even have a clue as to where to begin. (Not even the basics!) Some say that it's because our mothers never taught us how to manage money. Experts argue that maybe it's because of our lack of confidence; that we're terrified at trying a new lifestyle and think that it will cost more money to make new adjustments. So we become stuck in neutral.

Without getting knee-deep into psycho-social theory, let me just share what I think. The source of all this frustration might be nothing more than our emotional response to internal or external circumstances preventing us from reaching our goals. According to Jed Diamond, founder of *MenAlive,* an organization that helps men live healthier lives and author of *Male Menopause*, a man's frustration is usually increased when a goal is highly desirable (but unattainable) or we have overly optimistic expectations for reaching that unattainable, unrealistic or outlandish goal. We then retreat to our cave and deal with our frustrations through feeling burned out, fatigued, and depressed which in turn can result in aggressive behaviors and domestic strife.

This becomes especially difficult for male retirees who once were corporate hotshots and now find themselves feeling invisible, out-of the loop and in denial about their new identity and are too far above giving up their corporate lifestyle… downsizing their cell phones, giving up five dollar lattes and doing the day-to-day budgeting required of any normal person. Their frustration manifest themselves in the form of confusion, moodiness, feelings of unworthiness, inappropriate guilt, anger, impulsivity, alcohol abuse and carelessness with, or abuse of, prescription drugs. If you're experiencing these symptoms, find help fast by checking out the MenAlive website at Jed@MenAlive.com.

The Mars And Venus Conflict

Women, on the other hand, are living examples of human adaptability and strength. They appear to be more resilient to difficult conditions and don't get easily frustrated by conflicts, unrealized expectations, having to adjust to sudden, new situations and financial spikes in their lives. And do they process information differently? You bet they do. Genetic predisposition? Cortisol overload? Ask Mother Nature.

As John Gray asserts in his million dollar seller *Men Are From Mars, Women Are From Venus,* men and women are as different as creatures from another planet especially when communicating and during times of stress. Just like men demand to *withdraw* from time to time to a cave or their garage to focus (alone) on a solution to a problem, women demand to be heard from time to time preferably by a friend, a partner or a group to *process* options and solutions; a notion, according John Gray, males rarely understand. And therein lays the relationship challenges. One wants to process stuff and the other wants to fix stuff. Let's study a few other examples. I'm aware that I'm shamelessly cannibalizing parts of John's title and John, if you're reading this (as if!), we know what you've written are merely stereotypes and cannot be applied to everyone. Still, you've written a fun book.

Women Are From Venus (And That's Not All)

This was a man's world until Eve showed up. But let me just say that women are different…and smarter. They are psychic, walking think tanks. Why? Because from birth, they have been taught to be *process-based* thinkers and function on a spatial plane, thinking of everything at once from the moment they get up in the morning to the time they go to bed. Women use reasoning and logic better than men. "Now where in hell did you dig up the data that supports this generalization?" you ask. There are dozens of sources. For starters, you can Google it yourself or you can pick up John Gray's book to learn how to decode their behavior.

Women are given a glut of resources that outline techniques, standards and rules about shopping and saving money that even Alan Greenspan, the former chairman of the Federal Reserve, cannot touch. It's a damned art form. It comes as no surprise that women can make twenty dollars worth of groceries last a whole week, make bread taste like cake and (with a little mushroom gravy) make hamburger taste like steak. A woman who can cut corners and stretch a budget is looked upon with admiration and referred to as a minimalist, prudent, a wise spender, practical, economical, and a queen of thrift. Not only that, women know how to cut corners while still looking fashionable. Let me explain.

Women don't buy stuff just because it's cheap. There is a pathological joy attached to the hunt of a great deal. There is also a scientific cost analysis process attached to the art of buying, such as cost per wear…you know, how many times she can coordinate the outfit with other clothing items she already has socked away in her closet. Then, when planning the weeks menu, there is the number of servings per price calculations. (Most women cook, most men don't.) And when purchasing an automobile, fagetaboudit! That now requires an on-line consumer safety research project involving cost comparison data and gas mileage considerations then followed by focus group discussions to driving to the auto mall. It's mind boggling.

Men are from Mars (And your point?)

Men, as you have already guessed, can only process one thing at a time. We were born to solve things and mostly focus on a linear track. We think of work when working and we think of play when playing. And when it comes to fishing (or sex) we're oblivious to everything else.

We are not psychic mind readers and as a result some of us have to take special training just to decode women's behavior or be doomed to couples counseling for undetermined periods. We forget anything we said six months ago and therefore cannot defend ourselves when an issue that happened last May is brought up in November. Our mind lets us see only in six colors...much like Windows default on our computers. Peach and pumpkin, for example, are fruits, not colors. We have no idea what mauve is. If we happen to develop the slightest bit of sensitivity and ask our partner what's wrong and she says "nothing," we're going to believe it and act like nothing's wrong. We know she is lying, but it's just not worth the hassle pursuing. Besides, she will more than likely bring it up later, usually in the ear as we're driving to a function. And if she asks you if she looks fat (the universal trick question), just say "no" or you'll wind up sleeping on the couch that evening. But even that is okay. You see, for us, sleeping on the couch is like camping.

When men start to think of numerous things at once, and which may be totally unrelated to a task at hand, we are labeled ADHD. Copping to the lame excuse that we're multi-tasking (no doubt an activity invented by a woman) is not a window open to us. "What does all this psycho-babble mean and what does it have to do with my retirement?" you ask? I'm getting to it.

Let a man be careful with his spending and he is looked upon with disdain and considered a spendthrift, a tightwad, miserly and a penny pincher. If he is nearing retirement and desperately looking at ways to save a little dough, he is then labeled a "cheapskate." And when it comes to shopping, cooking and looking fashionable, fagetaboudit!

It is nearly impossible for us to be frugal and look fashionable. We buy an outfit because it covers us, protects us, and it's cheap. And if we like it, we wear it until it becomes threads. We wear two colors of socks, white and black all the time, all seasons. We never stop and analyze if that Hawaiian shirt, faded shorts, and sandals we bought at the swap meet even make a good fashion statement. And do we care?

When we're out buying an automobile, do we Google the latest consumer report and road safety data? I already know your answer. We'll take the red one with the 21-inch rims and the Bose system. Our mantra has been one of, "He who dies with the most toys wins." I have news for you. He who dies with the most toys is still DEAD nonetheless.

Here's my final, profound thought: I said earlier that men don't cook. We barbecue and we love it. Why? we get to be outside…one with the universe, scanning the evening stars searching for that universal Zen answer. Or maybe it's just another Neanderthal thing. Let's see. There's raw meat, sharp tools, flames, flammable liquids (whoosh!), smoke and beer. (Burping and farting outdoors is also fun for us.) What's not to like?

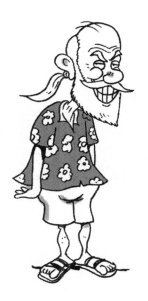

LIVING THE FRUGALISTA LIFESTYLE

Ten Zen Habits of a Frugalista

What does a retired frugalista know? How does he achieve financial security on a fixed income? What are his habits and how does one earn the right to be a part of his exclusive club called the *Buddhahood*? The answer is simple, yet complex. That is why it's called Zen. Relax. Take a deep breath and just let go. Look around you as you shop. What is he doing? The frugalista, I mean. Stop and talk to him. You'll find that he can be very approachable. A frugalista is always eager to share, to counsel, to point you toward *the* direction, the light…to move you from linear thinking to global thinking.

There are ten Zen habits that a frugalista adheres to in his search of the frugal lifestyle, some of which I am still trying to perfect daily and which may work for you as well. The habits include:

1. Never forgetting how your money was earned in the first place and how hard it is to keep.

2. Setting basic financial goals and sticking to them. I don't mean setting goals as it applies to future financial success. (You should have laid your nest egg twenty years ago.)

3. Saving and investing a small percentage of money each month, while focusing on your retirement future.

4. Developing one's imagination at all times. A frugalista is very spontaneous when money-saving opportunities arise.

5. Becoming a great networker. This is how a frugalista sniffs out new tips, ideas and locations for new bargains.

6. Creating a high sense of sociability. A frugalista is very social, and is not afraid to ask questions.

7. Being eager to help out a *newbie*. A frugalista will set you on the right path. All you have to do is ask. He may even invite you to join his *Buddhahood*, but only when he feels your spirit and mind are ready.

8. Never being afraid to ask for a discount. A frugalista saves hundreds (maybe thousands) of dollars yearly just by asking.

9. Saying "no" confidently (and comfortably). This is the easiest word in a frugalista's vocabulary.

10. Shopping wisely. A frugalista is not an impulsive shopper. He will never use a "sale" as a license to spend.

Zen is a discipline that teaches self-control and you already know how difficult it is to change old habits. Being a frugalista is like being a great dieter or bodybuilder. You can't crash diet or be sporadic in your workouts. The same applies to being frugal. You can't crash-save and expect positive results. You'll only lose your willpower and begin to binge-shop as you begin to get deeper in debt and become greatly disappointed. Sooner than later, you'll give up. Disappointment is something you don't need at this stage of your life.

Take things slow at first. Change is a constant daily personal evolution of discarding old habits and acquiring new ones and practicing them with great self-discipline. Steve Pavlina, author of *Personal Development for Smart People* writes that self-discipline has five pillars: Acceptance, Willpower, Hard Work, Industry, and Persistence. If you take the first letter of each word, you get the acronym "A WHIP", a cool way to remember that self-discipline means whipping yourself into shape.

Ready to give the frugalista lifestyle a shot? What follows are over one hundred ways to get started that come from my own personal fall-down-and-push-myself-up experiences. Learn what worked for me and with a little perseverance, could work for you. Zen teaches that perseverance is not a long race; it is many short ones…one after another. So take your time, be at one with it…have fun.

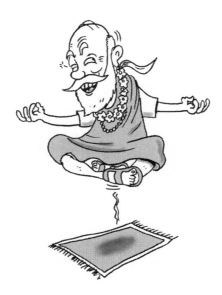

ZEN AND THE ART OF BUDGETING

"A fool and his money are soon partying."

No retired guy in his right mind would disagree when I say that debt is a dangerous game. Some people can succeed at it. The rest of us can't. It is what it is. People will also agree that budgeting your dollars is an important aspect of retirement. It is something that can no longer be delegated to a secretary like before, when you were the great Kahuna.

Running the Numbers

I know. I, too, hate the word *budget* because it strikes fear in my free-spending heart and blank stares from my male friends when I talk about it. So let's not call it a budget, but a *spending plan*. There. Feel better? No matter what name you give it, this still needs to get done in order to chart a proper course. First, be completely honest with yourself. Keep a record of how much you spend on a weekly basis. Then, each week thereafter, try to spend a little less than the week before. This can be a lot of fun as you start competing with yourself. You will be amazed how much lower you can go week by week, and how soon you will be known as "El Budgetista." Here's how you play:

- ***Switch your bank accounts*** if you're being charged maintenance fees. You shouldn't be spending your hard-earned money on extra charges. You should only be earning some serious interest on your checking and savings accounts.

- ***Record*** your income and expenses for a month. (You complained of nothing to do?) I'm going to assume you are organizationally challenged like me and so one month will be sufficient for now. But during that month, you will need to record every transaction that you make with your money. This is important. Use a pad or a spreadsheet, it doesn't matter.

- The important thing is that you record everything. Save all your receipts. Keep a record of where every penny goes. Be specific. Don't just write, "Spent $62 at Walmart." What exactly did you buy? This is important because the next month when you go shopping you may realize you didn't need the item you purchased last month (Ka-ching!).

- ***Scan your cancelled checks***. When doing this seemingly painful exercise, I was shocked at how much money was leaking out of my checking account. But that revelation made all that pain worthwhile. The first month I scanned my cancelled checks and learned I had spent $300 on eating out. I'm not kidding. I had no idea of the crap I was purchasing. At the end of the first month, rate your cancelled checks into two piles: 1) Things I needed to buy and 2) Things I could live without. You'll quickly get a snapshot of your spending habits. You'll soon begin to see the areas where you need work in curtailing your spending. The same can be done with your credit card statements.

- ***Write down*** income and necessary expenses. Assuming you live on a fixed income, write down the net (guaranteed) income you bring home every month, such as Social Security benefits, company retirement plan, etc. Cash in the bank does not count...ignore it and don't touch it. Next, list the mandatory things you know you need to pay over the course of a year.

Zen and The Art of Retirement

Use the information you collected during your first and second months of recording your expenses to help you with this. For variable bills, such as your electric and water bills, write down the average amount over the course of 12 months. Don't forget expenses that come up every quarter or twice yearly (property taxes), or only once a year such as insurance premiums and car registration renewal. Divide the total amount by the term covered, and enter that into your monthly expenses. If you pay your insurance every 6 months, divide the premium by 6, and that's the amount you're going to spend toward insurance every month. Finally, subtract all of your expenses from your income. The result may surprise you.

- **Adjust** your numbers as needed. If your income is greater than your expenses, that's fantastic! Take any extra income and put it toward your financial goals. This could be your emergency fund, debt repayment or a vacation...the possibilities are endless! In my case, a sinking feeling came over me as I concluded that my expenses were greater than my income. If this is you, there's no need to panic. You can fix it.

- **Slash** areas of your budget that are flexible. If you're spending $300 on eating out, that's a good place to start. The grocery bill is also very flexible. But be realistic. You have to eat. If you are having trouble making your income cover your expenses, and you can't cut expenses any further, you need to think about raising your income. Can you take on a part time job? Just know that you cannot continue to spend more than you earn. If you do, things will only get worse. Take whatever steps are necessary to get your spending level below your level of income, especially during your first year of retirement...the most critical time.

- **Torch** your credit cards. The Zen master teaches that when one is trying to get out of a hole, one must stop digging. If you can pay off all your credit cards except one that has a limit of less than $2000, you're practically out of the hole.

- ***Live by your plan***, but don't be too rigid. Once you have a budget in place, follow it. If you have already spent the $100 you budgeted for eating out for the month, don't spend any more. This is easier said than done, of course. I've screwed up many times. However, by keeping the budget in mind when you spend, you will continually move closer to your goals.

Now that you've gotten things into perspective and developed a savings plan, you can put your good decisions into action. Know that a budget isn't set in stone. You can adjust it if it's not working for you. The important thing is that you have started a plan. Without a plan your goals are just dreams (or nightmares).

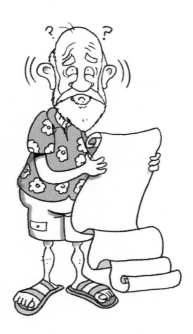

THE ZEN OF SHOPPING

"Veni, Vidi, Visa"
("I came, I saw, I charged it.")

Someone said, "If men enjoyed shopping, they'd call it research." Did you ever wonder why floor plans of supermarkets and department stores are changed so often? Call me insane, but I strongly believe that supermarkets and department stores are designed to cause bad karma. They are like casinos…they never want you to find your way out and are designed around manipulating, controlling, and profiting from human behavior.

I can picture in my mind a room full of management suits, sitting in a conference room with their liter mugs of "corporate crack" (coffee, with a depth charge of espresso) designing a mindless maze of floor plans while chuckling over the subliminal tricks they're pulling on the innocent shopper. Marketing studies show that shoppers are compulsive and can soon (unconsciously) memorize a routine and stick to the route where their weekly items are located, becoming oblivious to other products being marketed. But by turning the place upside down every couple of months it confuses the consumer's mind, forcing it to be introduced to thousands of new products we might have never noticed if the supermarket were left unchanged.

They know that as impulsive consumers, we will not resist buying several items we don't need as we search for those items on our list (Smell those pastries?) and before you know it, an hour and a half has been wasted as you find yourself at the front of the checkout line with this huge pyramid of junk in your cart that you didn't plan on buying. So what's your answer? You prepare by shopping purposefully.

Grab your highlighter. Here's how you begin:

Shop with a list. If you shop without a list, you may as well just throw your money away. Better yet, donate it to me. (I probably need it more than you.) Seriously, though, you need to prepare a list of everything you need, pulling from your weekly menu (you do make a weekly menu, don't you?) and checking to make sure you don't already have the items in your pantry, fridge or freezer. Make a "quick list" on a post-it note of things you are running low on and paste it on the fridge, adding to it so you have it handy when you go shopping. It is impossible for guys our age to remember what we ran out of at the end of the week. Do a "walk-around" your home before heading out to the store to make sure you're not forgetting anything.

Clean out your fridge. I'm not going to talk about this for very long. It's too gross. Don't you even care that you've got stuff growing in your fridge that is suddenly morphing from solids to liquids? Are you noticing that your leftovers have turned color and have begun to organize their own green political party? Toss them out and make room for the new, fresh stuff.

Eat what you have. A frugalista eats what he has first, thus cutting down on the amount of food he has to throw away and re-purchase.

Shop early weekend mornings. Why? It is a great thing to do when you feel out-of-sorts. Being around large stockpiles of food grounds you and makes you feel safe. Plus, there's something soothing about cruising around the aisles in the comfort of your favorite sweat pants. These are the best times to take your time and view all the discounts in peace and find some really great deals.

Never go for "one-item" trips. Leaving the house for one item wastes time and gas. And if you go to the corner Stop-N-Rob, you'll only get ripped off. Light bulbs, batteries, napkins, and general supplies can wait until you get to that great Dollar Store. For example, if a bulb burns out, go to another room in the house that has a two-bulb lamp on the ceiling and steal one. You'll make it until the next time you shop, plus you'll save electricity.

Buy Bulk. Go to Costco, Sam's Club or other bulk-purchase stores, grab a cart and go crazy. For example, the weekend is here and the best games will be on TV. Buy your beer and soft drinks by the case and make them last over a two-week period. Condition yourself to drink only two cans or less per day.

The same goes for chips and snacks. I find that buying a twenty four bag case of Cheetos or chips, and eating one small bag a day, are enough to quench my cravings for snacks. The same goes for meats. I learned this old trick of buying a family pack of pork chops (thin cuts), chicken drummettes, and hamburger patties, then separating them in Ziploc bags for individual servings and storing them in the freezer. This makes for a variety of delicious meals that can last for over a month. I could go on, but you've got the idea. Just get off the recliner and start exploring the possibilities.

Shop on a full stomach. This should be a no-brainer. Eat before going out the door to shop. Shopping with a full stomach prevents you from buying impulse items you will later regret. Eat a good meal first, and you'll be more likely to stick to your list... and spend less money. If you're going to a large bulk purchase store and are still hungry, start scarfing down the tons of free samples being offered...even if you don't like them.

Buy no-name brands. These days, there is very little difference in taste between generic and name brand foods. More and more stores are now contracting for "private label" products and selling them at much cheaper prices. There is a dollar difference in price between a bottle of Nyquil, the stuffy, sneezy, why is the room spinning medicine and the same product with the Target or Walmart name and you still get the same relief. Do the same when shopping for cereal, meats (No Name steaks), vitamins and soft drinks and you'll begin to see your grocery bill drop significantly. So what if the cute checkout girls at the register have identified you as *the cheapskate*? It's your money.

Don't buy junk food. Junk food not only costs a lot of money for about zero nutrition, it also makes you fat. Say nothing of the fact that junk food at your age will harden your arteries and possibly kill you. Is that what you want? Your goal is to eat and live a healthy lifestyle. Opt for fruits and veggies instead.

Shop the dollar stores. This is a secret guys know little about. You'd be surprised at the stuff you will find for a dollar at these great stores. They're a frugalista's paradise. The stigma of being viewed as poor or cheap has been removed by the quality of uniformly laid out décor and items of (sometimes) high-end overstocks that are being sold here. Dollar stores have great deals on generic brand grocery items, health and beauty products, over-the-counter medicines, household and cooking utensils.

Sign up for free customer rewards programs. Even if you rarely shop at the place being promoted, just having a rewards card for that place will eventually net you a ton of coupons and discounts.

Coupons are the way to go. "Isn't that a chick thing?" you ask? C'mon guys. You want free stuff don't you? Then start getting in touch with your inner chick. I can't say it enough. Coupons are the way to go. Today, there are coupons for literally everything. I can't believe I used to walk into a supermarket and pay full price for items that would have otherwise been discounted by just laying down a coupon on the conveyer belt. You don't have to cut coupons from the Sunday paper anymore. They're all online! It is so easy. Try these just for fun: www.registeredcoupons.com or www.thegrocerygame. com. Unless you're John McCain, everyone can use a computer these days.

Ask for the discounts. Many stores, hotels, restaurants, theaters and other establishments give senior citizen discounts, but seldom advertise or publicize them widely for obvious reasons. So you have to speak up. For example, the best time to attend a movie theatre is between 12:00 p.m. and 4:00 p.m. That is when the senior citizens score big time. And while you're there, don't forget to ask for the *kid's special* at the candy counter (that's if you forgot to bring your own treats). You'll get smaller portions and satisfy your cravings. Show me a retiree who eats a gallon tub of buttered popcorn and a liter of Pepsi and won't need an Emergency Medical Unit at the end of the movie. Even though you may have been trained in CPR, no one taught you how to use it on yourself.

Master the fifteen-day rule. If you're a *must-have* ADD retiree like me, whenever you're considering making an unnecessary purchase, wait fifteen days and then ask yourself if you still want that item. Quite often, you'll find that the feeling to buy will pass and you'll have saved yourself some money by simply waiting.

Master the ten-second rule. Whenever you're grocery shopping and pick up an item that is not on your list, pause for ten seconds and ask yourself why you're buying it and whether you actually need it or not. If you can't find a good answer, put the item back. It's quite simple and after a little practice...Ka-ching!

Look for used stuff first. Guys are the first to grab the first thing that looks good and take it home. (Some marry in the same manner!) If you need something, I mean really need it, not just want it, see if someone you know has one that they don't use or need anymore. Send out an email to family or friends, or just ask around. You might be surprised. I was about to buy a printer, and then found out my daughter had just bought a laser printer and didn't need her old inkjet printer anymore. I snagged it and saved a whopping $100. If you are new to the Internet, you may want to explore Craigslist.com or freecycle.org for good used items. Get out of the house and visit garage sales. Better yet, estate sales are the new "bang." You can find just about anything you need, from electronics, to books, to furniture and tools. Everything! You get to socialize a bit, meet some nice people and perhaps find that special item you have been looking for.

Invest in a crock-pot. Odds are that you are already on the cardiologist diet (if it tastes good spit it out). A crock-pot is perhaps the best money-saving deal on the planet and the healthiest way to cook delicious meals. You can just dump in your ingredients in the morning, put it on simmer, and dinner is done when you get home. You can then store the leftovers in Ziploc bags for quick dinners in the future. There are countless recipes out there for all varieties of health conscious foods, and every time you cook this way, you're saving money.

Don't spend a ton of money entertaining grandchildren. You will find that children enjoy the simple things and just being with you. Go to a large grocery or appliance store and ask them for a couple of large empty boxes so when your grandkids visit you, you can build them a cool fort. Throw in their sleeping bags and they will be chomping at the bit for the next sleepover at grandpa's house. I have learned that kids can destroy toys within 24 hours after they get them, but a fort can last forever (in their memories, for sure).

Lose the health club. Admit it. You rarely go to your health club and are wasting $60 per month. Just break loose and take a brisk walk or a jog each evening. You can buy a huge exercise ball that you can use for sit-ups (and won't damage your back) and some light muscle exercises right at home. These exercises can be done at home for very little and the health benefits are enormous.

Cell phone: your must have lifeline. "But I can't afford the charges." you say? All is not lost. Samsung has come up with the cell phone answer for seniors. Have you heard of the *"Jitterbug?"* It is a phone that is easy to use and includes immediate, friendly, helpful service.

There are no gimmicks, no contracts to sign, and no roaming charges within the U.S. It is slightly larger than a regular cell phone and with ring tones that don't sound like frogs on crack. It comes backlit, with larger buttons and text. And finally they have provided us with powerful speakers that are louder. All this and for about ten bucks a month. They will also provide you with 24-hour link to Jitterbug operators that can make calls for you in an emergency, provide directory assistance and add names to your phone list. The next time you're at the mall, talk to the kid in the cell phone kiosk.

AARP has your back. *The American Association of Retired Persons* (AARP) offers its members a wide variety of discounts on travel, auto rental, insurance, and anything else sold in the United States. But none of these advantages will come to you automatically. The astute furgalista has to make himself aware of these opportunities by asking, applying for them, and by learning how to use them daily.

Avoid buying into get rich schemes. You want to reach *Buddhahood?* Then stop wasting your hard-earned money in get rich schemes. Crap in a gilded cage is still crap. Look, you're not going to bring in any more income than what you already have. You have now made a serious commitment to live (and well) within your means. Let me share with you the top twelve biggest wastes of money. See if you've done any of these and if you have, stop it. You're spinning your wheels, man.

Top twelve wastes of money and time:

There are twelve things a frugalista does not do. These give out bad karma and empty your wallet.

1. Buying lottery tickets every time you gas up at the local Stop-N-Rob. Only people who don't need money win lotteries. (Or so it seems.)

2. Buying anything (except coffee or gas) at the local Stop- N-Rob. Coffee is a *loss leader* and studies show that a shopper at a Stop-N-Rob will (almost always) purchase other items in addition to the coffee. Buyers beware.

3. Buying food at the movies or ball games. Bring your own stash. (But you knew this already.)

4. Taking action on *hot* investment tips. (There's a sucker born every minute.)

5. Paying an annual fee on credit cards (and I hope you only have one card that is well hidden).

6. Shopping at high-end clothing stores. T-shirts and underwear come in packs of six at Target, Kmart and Walmart. A couple of packs of each should last you a long time. (Recycle the old ones as cleaning cloths.)

7. Paying fees for your checking accounts.

8. Buying car dealer extras.

9. Shopping on QVC or the Home Shopping Network.

10. Keeping the bulk of your money in interest-bearing savings accounts.

11. Buying extended warranties on electronics and appliances.

12. Paying full retail on anything. Hold off until the holiday sales. Any frugalista knows that everything can be had wholesale… or pretty close to it.

If you can avoid these twelve traps in your retirement, you will be known as a frugalista. I guarantee it. All you need to do is assess and adjust your spending habits (and attitudes) and determine how much you need to comfortably give up while living the happy, frugal lifestyle. It's all about using common sense when spending your money. Remember, common sense and good humor will make your retirement a walk in the park.

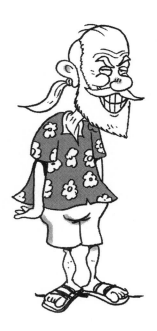

THE ZEN OF EATING OUT
A LA CHEAP

"If you can get nothing better out of the world, get a good dinner out of it, at least."

In the first place, a bottle of wine and a sixteen ounce steak at your age went out with your bell bottom pants and wide ties. It's now about savoring what you eat and being mindful of your health. That said:

- **There is a free lunch (sometimes).** In 2001, I was between jobs and had $60 to my name. My bank had a special deal where if you used the ATM at the Super America convenience store, you could get a free hot dog and a soda pop for each transaction you made. For lunch, I'd go to one convenience store, withdraw $20, and get a free hot dog and soda pop. Then I'd go to another convenience store for dinner, withdraw another $20 and get another hot dog and soda pop. I'd then go to my bank, re-deposit the $40 and start the whole scene the next day. It kept me fed for quite a while. I wasn't cheap; I was broke.

- **Order side items.** Is it my imagination, or do buffalo wings taste like chicken? Anyway, a salad and an appetizer can often make for a delicious but affordable meal. If you must drink, go for one glass of wine.

- **Join a dining club.** There are a boatload of "two for one" offers from restaurants that are ready to give you a free entrée when you order a second one. This is also a great way to try new restaurants.

- **Dinner date?** You don't have to order two dinners. It is more cost effective (and romantic) to order one dinner you both like and split it. Spend the savings on a glass of wine for each of you. Restaurants typically serve way too much food anyway and if you try to finish a large meal, you'll both be so bloated with gas neither of you will be in a mood for a sleepover. Know what I mean?

- **Restaurant coupons.** Check your Sunday paper. There are several restaurant coupons scattered throughout that can save you serious dough.

- **Go for breakfast or lunch specials.** Lunch specials are way cheaper than dinners, and breakfasts are generally even cheaper. Always ask about the senior or the daily special, as it can often be a good deal. As you are close to finishing your meal ask for a refill of your coffee or tea. Finish your meal, and then just before you get ready to pay, ask for a Styrofoam cup for your drink so that you have something to sip on the way to your destination. Clever? Of course.

- **Order water.** You didn't drive to your favorite restaurant for the liquor or soft drinks. So when you order that great meal, wash it down with a nicely chilled glass of tap *agua.*

- **Skip dessert.** At fancy restaurants, desserts are a rip off. But you knew that already.

- **Happy Hour.** Right on! *Two-fers* (two-for-one) are always offered at your favorite pub along with snacks and appetizers that can (sometimes) serve as a meal.

- **Fast foods are in again (sort of).** Fast foods are becoming healthier. I was in Wendy's the other day and had a fantastic Chinese chicken salad. Subway and other sandwich places that are also offering healthier options. Stay away from those quadruple by-pass Mexican places that sell burritos the size of your thigh. They are too expensive and, in time, will kill you.

- **Do lunch instead.** If you want a fine meal, visit your favorite restaurant near the end of lunchtime. They serve the same specials, but in smaller portions and for cheaper prices and they will hold you past dinner.

ZEN AND THE ART OF COOKING (AND SEX)

"I cook, therefore I am."

Now that I have your attention, let me plant this little seed and maybe you will nurture it and let it grow. Learning to cook can be a spiritual and healthy thing to do (especially in retirement). In fact, for me, the kitchen has become my Zen temple. It is where I am oblivious to everything, deeply breathing in the aromas and being one with the stove, the knife and my large wooden spatula. (Why wood?)

Tai Chi in the kitchen

Most men grow up without being encouraged to cook, and in adulthood, most quickly find someone else to do it for them. It is little wonder that as a guy, you may first find the task of cooking as a bothersome obstruction to the mind and senses. That's a shame, because cooking can be a great form of meditation. Cooking is a way of leaving the struggle and a getting into the moment.

Even though you're retired, it's still a jungle out there and some days you just have to say, "Screw this" and make more time for things that bring you peace. That is the paradox of Zen. It teaches that by letting stuff go, one finds what one needs. Cooking does that for me. It is a way of losing oneself. It has no right or wrong answers. Cooking just is...a Zen feel. Allow me to show you the true path of culinary enlightenment.

Clean and free your mind. Begin using the act of cooking as a Zen art form...a kind of Tai-chi exercise performed in creative solitude. Find the mellow jazz cuts on that iPod your kids gave you for Christmas, sip a little wine and practice this every time you cook. Soon you will learn to free your mind and let go of the day-to-day clutter and begin taking more time for joy.

Unless you are neurotic, you cannot cook and think about your job, money and paying bills all at the same time while chopping, slicing, mixing, spicing, beating, whipping, combining, measuring, cutting, pouring, tasting, sautéing and stirring. You are in your Zen zone... lost in the present. Being lost in the present can be a wonderful state of mind for a anyone. It is like crawling inside this tiny zone in your brain where, with a little practice, you learn to park your consciousness. It's like giving it a well-deserved "time out." Sipping that wine, prepping the food, stirring and taking in those mystical aromas from the cilantro and garlic puts you *there*. If you just let things be, you will soon become the food and the food will become you.

The Zen of sharing

If you have someone special in mind to share this miracle with then you have been truly blessed. Sharing food is an ancient form of bonding. It is about the sensual excitement brought on by the subtle aromas of specially selected spices and the peace and contentment you find in the mixing of disparate ingredients into one miraculous whole...then sharing it with someone special.

If I were to ask you where the most romantic place in the home is, you'd more than likely respond, "the bedroom." You are so not right! Assuming you want to interact with someone special in your retirement years and assuming you hate hanging out in bars picking up *sex care providers,* let's talk about the romance that can be created in the kitchen when cooking for someone special.

First, should an attractive honey accept your invitation to a home cooked meal, consider yourself blessed by the gods. Second, you are probably thinking, "How in the hell can I get into my Zen state with this beautiful woman in my kitchen? It just won't work here."

I feel your mental anguish. How can you get in your Zen zone when you're trying to make small talk, while wondering if sex will be on her agenda tonight and if you're going to be personally involved…while cooking at the same time? That is too powerful a concept for the male brain. Take a deep breath and find your quiet place, while I enlighten you.

Women enjoy having a man cook for them, plain and simple. They feel they are being nourished by your kindness. For some it's erotic…a form of foreplay. (I don't have the research to prove this, but I think you're safe.) If you worked doubly hard to get that gorgeous someone to come to your home in the first place, you had better make a good impression. Learn to cook…anything. But keep it simple. Preparing food for an upset stomach is not very romantic. Stick to appetizers followed by a light meal at first. The presentation of your meal is more romantic than the content. Strawberries, chocolate and maybe some exotic cheeses with some great wine are a few choices that work. That can then be followed up with a light chicken or fish. But focus on presentation at all times.

You want to make a good impression so as to insure a return visit, but having a woman sitting on a barstool in your kitchen sipping a glass of your best box wine can be daunting. Having her watch you cook as you make up cute distracting jokes while trying to look down her blouse without her catching you is taking multi-tasking to its highest level. We're still prone to a state known as *tit madness* that puts all men, regardless of age, into a mild stupor, making us disoriented and distracted from the task at hand.

So you try to focus on monitoring the simmering peas on the stove, and answering questions about the pictures pasted on your fridge, as you incoherently babble about how, back in the day, you helped Bill Gates invent the PC. You think to yourself, "What do you do now, stud?"

Don't fret. I've got the answer that will make you the Zen stud of your condo complex. First of all, conversing while a man cooks is erotic to many women. I don't have the data to support this, but I think the odds are still in your favor. Second, to some women klutzy guys are cute (sprinkle a little flour around the kitchen). And third, women love to process crap men don't even bother thinking about. (I don't know if that's true, but I have a hunch.) So, before you pick up your club, Mr. Flintstone, you've got to learn to do all three. Once you do, and can process intently without collapsing, you're in the Zen zone, my man.

Before the meal is even ready to eat, you'll find that she has suddenly moved closer behind you with a warm strange grin on her face. Do you know the look that women give when they want to have sex? Neither do I. Still, you inconspicuously turn off the burner, and say to yourself, "This is it." Horny Zen Masters refer to this altered state as a *transcendent communion*...the state that surpasses the passions of the flesh. (Riiight!)

The truth is you already know in advance that you've got at least ten minutes left on the Shake-N-Bake chicken in the oven and the three-day Cialis you took two hours ago should just about kick in. And as she takes that big wooden spatula from your hand and rips off your apron, you find you are both in transcendent communion...at one with the universe. If that isn't nirvana, then someone please tell me what is?

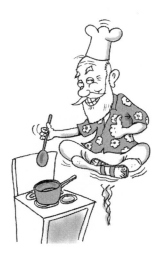

RECIPES OPEN THE DOOR

(But you must enter alone.)

The Zen of ethnic cooking

To taste is to believe. There exist hundreds of easy-to-prepare recipes that can be used in retirement. But none match the Zen created by ethnic cooking (Greek, Italian, Middle Eastern, Mexican…no matter) and the wonderful aromas that can permeate your home and announce to your guests, "Welcome, pull up a plate."

Ethnic cooking does that for many people. It can be a great form of meditation and relaxation. It is simple process (or our grandmothers wouldn't do it) that can impress the best of discriminating chefs. Cooking with herbs and spices makes a dish complete and places you in the ranks of Emil Lagasse (maybe). No matter what you cook, there have to be the magic ingredients of cilantro, garlic, onions, cumin, curry, ginger and others that make your olfactory senses snap to attention. Spices can also affect relationships. Masters teach that we can bring out the best in ourselves by bringing out the best in the dishes we prepare. Guys, highlight this little gem. Ethnic cooking has been known to change relationships from stagnant and stale to spicy and hot. The kitchen is the first erogenous zone. If you don't know what the others are, then cooking is not your problem.

Cooking with spices also makes you a creative genius. There are no right or wrong answers. The recipes are merely guidelines. Mom never used them. And what is great is that you can add more pinches of this or that (usually from a two-foot distance for drama) in order to bring out the personality of the masterpiece you are creating and while being admired by those around you. There are particular spices that an ethnic kitchen cannot do without.

Though I have two drawers full of all types of spices, my must-have-from-the-get-go spices include:

- All-spice (ground)
- Ginger(powdered)
- Salt, pepper
- Cumin
- Chili powder
- Spanish tarragon (for lamb)
- Lemon extract
- Cinnamon (ground)

- Red pepper (ground)
- Steak rub
- Oregano (Italian and Greek)
- Vanilla extract
- Curry powder
- Cloves
- Ginger root
- Nutmeg

Move over, Emil Lagasse. But I must tell you, don't think that you can throw something in a pan, cover it up and then go watch TV. Good ethnic cooking requires (even demands) monitoring, tasting, stirring and adding the ingredients as you are cooking (a spiritual Tai chi). Zen Masters teach that often the *answers* we seek are right before us, yet people seek them in all the wrong places. I have come to learn that the spirituality one seeks is sometimes no further away than the bowl in front of you. Whoa!

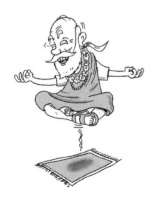

It's all up to you now

The title suggests that recipes open the door, but you must enter alone. It is for this reason that I have laid the groundwork for what could be years of exciting cooking experiences in your retirement. I have provided for you some great websites that can quickly get you on the road to being the Zen master of your kitchen. They include:

- www.cdkitchen.com
- www.betterrecipes.com
- www.culinarycafe.com
- www.spiceadvice.com
- www.gourmetslueth.com
- www.cyberspacegrill.com
- www.cheapcooking.com
- www.thecheapbook.com
- www.ezinearticles.com
- www.campbellkitchen.com
- www.recipesearch.com

The sites above have been reviewed and are some of the best recipe sites on the net for male-targeted cooking. Please contact the sites individually if you don't find the particular food or ingredients you need. Bon appetit!

THE ZEN OF ROMANCING ON-THE-CHEAP

"Focus. The 'right' one may be right beside you."

We spend most of our time searching for the right person. Zen suggests that we stop running around seeking and begin seeing what is right in front of our eyes. Look at a person who is close to you right now - anyone it happens to be. Notice the subtle ways in which you push each other away. Stop doing that. Allow the two of you to be together in whatever way you are. Let all of it be fine just as it is. Zen also teaches that neither romance nor your spirit dies at retirement. When was the last time you and your significant other put on a pair of tennies and kicked it around the neighborhood? When was the last time you praised your partner? Try it, even if it frightens her at first. When was the last time you helped her around the house or left her a love note? These are all natural gifts we can give each other. Look, no husband has ever been shot while vacuuming or washing dishes. Start giving naturally. I have listed for you many ways that a retired male can score with his partner. It does not have to be fancy or expensive, just something that will add to her day.

I believe that the golden rule of writing requires that if I like a piece of work, I must share it and its author with other people who like it...not because of copyright laws (though important), but because I am too lazy to recreate something that someone has already done well. Richard Stallman author of *Zen Habits* kindly allowed me to review his forty romantic ideas and pick my favorite twenty-five (some of which I've already used with great success). If you want to score a touchdown with your partner, these twenty five tips will get you to the five-yard line. Pick the five that you like and do them on a regular basis without expecting something in return. There'll be cookies and milk nightly, I guarantee it. And you don't have to spend a fortune doing it:

1. Make friends with yourself. Accept yourself unconditionally. Stop judging and rejecting yourself. Be still; look within. Then make a change and your partner will appreciate the difference.

2. Cook a romantic dinner. The kitchen is the first erogenous zone. (If you don't know the others, then cooking is not your challenge.)

3. Take massage lessons together and then give yourselves a full-body massage.

4. Go to a hot yoga class together.

5. Pack a Sunday picnic and take a ride to the ocean or lake.

6. Burn a CD of her favorite love songs and listen to them over a bottle of her favorite wine.

7. Snuggle together under a blanket, on the sofa, on a rainy day and read a book to each other.

8. Send her a love email every week.

9. Buy her flowers monthly.

10. Snuggle together while watching romantic movies.

11. Get a bottle of wine and sit out on the porch and star gaze.

12. Bring home good coffee or a decadent sweet.

13. Take a walk down memory lane — visit some of the special places from your early days of dating.

14. Go antique shopping and enjoy a luncheon.

15. Take walks in the rain.

16. Bring home great take-out, and light some candles.

17. Have a pizza picnic in front of your warm fireplace.

18. Slow dance to the oldies.

19. Take a nap together. Why do you think they call it "afternoon delight?"

20. Make a list of everything you love about her and mail it to her.

21. Take some quiet time and talk about your day.

22. On Sunday morning, make a fruit plate and coffee and bring it (along with her favorite section of the newspaper) up to the bedroom.

23. Surprise her with an evening ride to the river, spread a blanket and uncork a bottle of wine.

24. Grab some good wine and have a candlelight dinner on the patio.

25. Save the leftover wine for the next day. Leftover wine???? Hello!!!!!!!!

This is not deep stuff. When you're not in love, something's the matter, plain and simple. Don't let anyone tell you that losing interest in romance and sex is a natural part of aging. I'm here to testify that sex after sixty is great. A bit slower, but great nonetheless. Give these twenty-five tips a try. You're still the man!

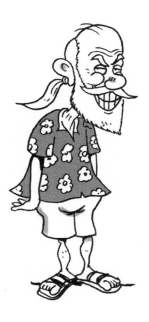

HOME IS WHERE THE ZEN IS

"The more out of the box, the more in your wallet."

If having to become organized makes you shudder, then this chapter is not for you. Face it, home is where the Zen is. Your home is your Zen temple. So it's time to step back and take a good look at your surroundings. What's going on? Does your home look like a nuclear fall out? Is it so cluttered and dusty that when your grandkids visit they write messages on the furniture? Where can you go to decompress?

I know from experience that clutter in a home can collect faster than a flock of seagulls around a discarded bag of French fries. I also know from experience that physical clutter breeds mental clutter and mental clutter results in chaos in your daily living...something you don't need at this stage of your life. Ask yourself, "Is my home conducive to living a Zen-like life?" I don't mean lighting incense and chanting around the house in a robe and sandals. The home needs to be a place that allows you to live a calmer life. It must be infused with a sense of peace...a feeling of *rightness*. It must be a place where you can rise above those feelings of confusion, fear, and anxiety one gets by what's going on in the outside world. Begin to unclutter your home and mind. It's time for that spring cleaning I talked about chapters ago. The more you get rid of the clutter, the greater peace you will find. At this stage of your life, clutter is not your friend.

Zen creativity also begins in the home. Creativity and the frugal lifestyle are equal Zen concepts. Both fit the conditions for creativity. On one hand, being a frugalista inspires us to become creative.... and on the other hand, a little creativity can result in living a happy, frugal lifestyle. The more you think out of the box, the more money you can put in your wallet.

Just don't get yourself all worked up. You're new lifestyle isn't that difficult to organize. But it's going to take you a while to get to our level of skill...a Zen master.

In this section, I have included some sensible money-saving tricks that put money in your wallet. I don't know about you, but it is nearing winter and I'm already planning for that trip to Mexico. So let's begin with winter savings tips first.

Declutter

Your home is your (Zen) temple. Keep it clean and organized. I find it pretty amazing when I go through my closets and garage and see all the crap I bought over a period of time and it's an even more gratifying process to get rid of all the junk, making me realize how useless all our consumer shopping is. I don't need any of the stuff anymore! You will especially enjoy the peace, joy and sense of accomplishment that decluttering provides.

Winterize

Unless you live on the west coast or in the deep south, for many of us the chill in the fall air reminds us that it is time to *winterize*. (Minnesota-speak for: "That damn, cold, white shit will soon be covering my driveway.") I always freak out around this time of year because I just know that we'll have a bitter winter of such a magnitude that it shrinks the bravest Scandinavian's testicles. Say nothing of the agony brought on by spending three months sadly staring out the window sipping brandy as the bulk of my hard earned money is being used to heat my leaky home.

Northerncheapskate.com and www.cheapskatemonthly.com are valuable resources that people in cold climates tap into yearly. I recommend these sites for their reliability in providing money saving tips that easily redirect money into your pocket and not up the chimney. It is called *winterizing:*

1. Check furnace and hot water boiler. Change any filters and make sure the chimney is clean. This is also a good time to check those smoke detector and carbon monoxide detector batteries.

2. Seal up those leaks. Get down to the local discount hardware store and buy some weather stripping and caulk.

3. Wrap your windows. If you're in an old house with old windows, you can get plastic wrap to cover them. It's not an attractive look, but it does save energy. Use insulated curtains to block out the cold at night.

4. Install a programmable thermostat. Turn down the thermostat. Just a few degrees can mean a 10 percent decrease in your heating bill. If your house has different zones, keep the lower level a little warmer than upstairs. Heat rises, so take advantage of it! If you will be leaving for more than an hour, turn down the thermostat.

5. Wear sweaters and slippers. I'm amazed when people complain about how expensive their heat bill is while running around in short sleeves and bare feet. Turn down the heat and wear a sweater and a pair of klunky slippers.

6. Invite some friends over. Learn to make soups and collect wines and invite your friends over. The more the merrier! Ask them to bring a special wine they like and ask them to discuss the wine with the group. This always makes for a lot of fun conversation.

7. Kill-A-Watt. (Get it?) Replace those incandescent bulbs with compact fluorescents. You'll save money on your electric bill.

Buys in the 'hood

Life is good! Garage sales are a great way to pass the time. Some people just don't understand the Zen of garage or estate sales. The Zen, my friend, is not in getting that antique Lone Ranger alarm clock from the 1950's or that mint condition album of the Beatles' *Hard Days Night,* but in the hunt for the deal and the entire day spent outdoors in the sunshine with people you want to spend time with. On the other hand, since we've already talked about decluttering, you can empty your closets and garage of all the junk you've collected (and will never use) and have your own sale. The Zen of having your own sale is putting out a sign that says something like, "Please buy my crap!" Pull up a comfortable canvas back chair and see how easily you will meet some of the greatest people while making a few bucks in the process.

The Zen of duct tape

Before you read any further, ask yourself, "Do I really want to know this?" Someone (probably famous) once said, **"Duct tape is like the** *force*: It has a dark side and a light side and it holds the universe together." This is not new. Guys like us know more than 1,000 uses for duct tape.

Duct tape is gender neutral and, with a little creativity, can be used by both men and women to mend, paste, reattach, repair and even cover your grandson's mouth when he's crying because the kids left him with you too long. This stuff is a thing of beauty (all silvery) and works on everything. No need to spend your hard-earned money at Target. What you need around the home is as close as your toolbox. If you haven't figured it out already, some great uses for duct tape include: hanging posters, decorating book covers, fixing broken tail lights, taping wires, repairing cracked windshields, patching rips in your favorite winter jacket, repairing broken garden hoses, repairing torn pillows, mending furniture, taping cuts and bruises, repairing rips in a shower curtain and even taping together that cardboard fort you'll be building for the grandkids. You see now? All that money you'll be saving by using duct tape will get you that "super-sized" value meal the next time you go to Burger King.

Trash the TV

I've heard that in California people don't throw their garbage away. They just recycle it into television shows. That's not true. But there isn't anything on television that is of real value. In case you didn't know, the word *television* is half Greek and half Latin. What creative good can come from that? Back in the day we only had four channels of crap. Today, we have 166 channels of the same recycled *doo doo*. There is nothing wrong with watching two to three hours (spread out) of TV per day. Any more than that, you might as well dig a hole and throw dirt over yourself.

One big way to save money is to watch less television. There are a lot of financial benefits to this: less exposure to guilt-inducing ads, more time to focus on other things in life, lower electrical bills and so on. Retiring happy is getting out and finding creative, challenging things to do. TV is the easiest form of entertainment and doesn't require much energy or creativity, which is why people do it. Not to bum you out, but TV is a medium that allows millions of people to laugh at the same time and still remain lonesome. If you can't trash it, then at least cut down on it.

The Zen of an organized kitchen

"Waste not, want not" is the frugalista's code. Nothing could be truer in these trying times. We're all feeling the pinch. Costs consistently creeping upward, gasoline prices have gone through the roof and do we dare discuss our skyrocketing grocery bills? What's next?

There's one benefit that most guys don't understand for having an organized kitchen and that is saving money. What? Hold on. The connection between having an organized kitchen and saving money is not immediately obvious to us. But think about it. A disorganized kitchen can hide smaller expenses that add up in the long run. For example, a disorganized kitchen causes us to view cooking as a big hassle (we can't find anything) so we get lazy and eat out instead. Have you scanned your cancelled checks or your credit card statements lately? How much are you spending on eating out? Don't bother. I already know your answer.

Cooking in an organized kitchen allows you to see your whole inventory (spices, refrigerated goods, supplies) so that you don't have to duplicate anything. When you begin utilize the foods which before were being pushed to the rear of the fridge, you begin to save a little money by avoiding waste and reducing costly trips to the doctor because you're eating healthier.

Go through all the stuff in the kitchen and throw out anything you don't use on a regular basis, especially if you're now living in a small condo or apartment. This is the hardest part because the frugalista in you will want to keep everything.

1. Separate bulk meats into Ziploc bags. Then as you prepare for a meal, you merely take out a bag, thaw it and cook it. I buy the packs of thin sliced pork chops, chicken and hamburger or steaks (5 oz. portions) and separate them into Ziplocs by portions. You can then thaw out a package as needed. Don't forget to look for the sales and then stockpile those bad boys for the winter.

2. Separate your pizza. When the Pizza Hut has their sales, buy the family size, eat a couple of slices then divide it into pairs. Place each pair in Ziplocs then freeze them for other days. No need to pig out. Your goal is to satisfy your appetite.

3. Cook enough food for two meals. Leftovers are cheaper than shopping for entire new meals.

4. Use more potatoes with your meals. They are inexpensive and offer a great deal of nutrition. A cheapskate retiree has to be creative. For example, I like to bake a potato then top it with

melted cheese and bacon bits. Chase it down with a glass of your finest Pinot Noir... nirvana!

5. Buy generic brands. There is little difference between generic and name brand.

6. Goodwill and Salvation Army stores can be a great place for a cheapskate retiree to grab some great deals. There are some great casual wear items for pennies on the dollar. Try to avoid those selling bell bottom pants and leisure suits. (Need I explain?)

7. Avoid the expensive skinless chicken. You'll save more by buying regular chicken breasts, skinning them yourself and saving dollars. Or buy chicken drummettes for even less money... with a little Cajun sauce, they are to die for.

8. Cut back on meat consumption. Make one meal a week meatless such as veggie pizza, a quiche, or quesadillas. Try using less meat than a recipe calls for. If a recipe calls for 1 lb of ground beef, try to use a 1/2 lb instead. You're only after the flavor, anyway.

9. Unless you are living in Mexico, don't recycle the plastic bottled water empties. Refill them from the sink and reuse them. These days, tap water is very healthy, tastes just as good as bottled water and is just as wet.

10. Save all shopping bags and use them for trash can liners. (But you knew this already.)

11. Shop at bakery outlets...every city has one. Day-olds are the new "fresh."

12. Don't empty coffee filters daily. Replace them every other day. Just add half the amount of fresh coffee to the already existing coffee filter. One sip and you'd think you were camping in the hills of Montana.

13. Plant a victory garden in a planter on your porch. Recycle the coffee grounds on top as mulch.

The Zen of an organized bathroom

I like learning new stuff and applying it in my daily living. These are a few things I have learned about having an organized bathroom and have found that it's saving me money.

1. Get thee to Costco or Sam's Club and buy bulk. There are great bargains in bathroom tissues, hand soaps, sanitizers, toothpastes, shampoo, bodywash and bathroom cleaner. By buying bulk, you'll always have what you need and will save a ton of money.

2. Change that shower head. Did you know that showers consume more than 20% of all the water used indoors? They use more hot water than any appliance in the house. Installing a low-flow shower head can cut your water and heating bill by one-third.

3. Fix that leaking toilet. Why do we enjoy jiggling the toilet handle instead of merely replacing the unit inside for just twelve bucks? A running toilet can use as much as 2000 gallons of water a year, doubling your monthly water bill.

4. Turn off the water while shaving and brushing your teeth. When you're ready to rinse, turn it back on.

5. Keep one toothbrush. Why do guys have more than one toothbrush in their dispenser? Do we have lots of group sex? I doubt it. So why do we need four?

6. Invest in a toilet brush and a little Spic and Span. I don't know how this saves money, but a clean bathroom makes for a healthy living environment and not a castle of biological horrors. Oh, don't store the toilet brush with the toothbrushes.

7. Shampoo can last forever (or so it seems). When your shampoo gets half empty, pour a little water in it to extend shampoo life for a few more weeks. When you're through, recycle the bottle. It's not a collector's item.

8. Don't skimp on toilet paper. Buy bulk, and guys, I won't spend too much time on this one. Buy the good, thick (the one with the dancing bears) toilet paper. It's worth every penny. You wind up using twice of the one-ply cheap stuff anyhow and those can cause wiping accidents. (No need to get graphic.)

9. Use baking soda instead of toothpaste, except when you have a special guest for a sleepover. Then bring out the good stuff. (See section on baking soda in next chapter.)

10. Partied all night? Bags under your eyes? Not a problem. Eliminate puffiness by dabbing a little Preparation H under each eye. Prep H is a *vasoconstrictor* that instantly relieves swelling under the eyes…and other places.

11. Replace your shaving razor only when it begins to draw blood and exposes your inner muscles (usually every two months). Never leave your razor lying around looking like a prop of a Sweeny Todd play.

12. Cure for common headache. Who needs aspirin? When life gives you lemons (or limes), grab the Tequila. Take a lime, squeeze it in some Tequila. Chill for two minutes, then drink it. Works for me.

LIFE ON THE CHEAP

"If you loan someone $20 and never see that person again, it was probably a good investment."

Life-on-the-cheap can be over the top at times. Living within your means doesn't mean that you have to do without. It just means that you need to look at your money in a different way. If you can keep that dollar in your pocket awhile longer and seek other ways to make your resources stretch, then why not? Below are some creative (no, bizarre) cheapskate lifestyle tips I have received from folks in our *Buddhahood.* I'd be selective about which ones to use, but they are all worth mentioning, if at least for the chuckles.

1. Use peroxide to take out a food stain in your clothes before washing them. The peroxide breaks down the protein in the stain so that it will come out in the wash. Taking bloodstains out of your white shirt is another matter (and a pretty violent image). At your age, if you've got a T-shirt with blood all over it, maybe laundry isn't your biggest problem, big guy.

2. Adjust the temperature in the house to two settings: one for the day and one for the evening. It accounts for half of your utility bill. Check out comparefurnace.com for more tips.

3. Don't toss your $125.00 wing tip shoes. Double the life of your shoes by re-heeling them for thirty bucks.

4. Use one bulb in a two bulb lamp. How much light do you need?

5. Buy same color socks. I have ten pairs of black and ten pairs of white athletic socks. (Nobody really uses brown, anymore.) If one gets worn or lost I just pull another sock out of the drawer and move on down the road.

6. Give holiday presents from the dollar store. Your relatives know you're on a fixed income. And what about those ties they've been giving you the past forty years? (For once, why can't gift-giving be retaliatory?)

7. Hold potlucks. Having relatives over for the holiday dinner? Have a potluck instead of an elaborate feast. Everyone knows you're on a budget. By having everyone bring something, it cuts your workload and grocery bill in half.

8. Look for the two-fers (two-for-one deals). Magazines and museums, in particular, often try to extend their audience by having current customers hook up their friends with a free subscription or membership.

9. Don't renew magazine subscriptions right away. The longer you wait, the cheaper the offers to renew.

10. Need towels? Wait until the swim season is over and go to your local YMCA or high school and ask them for the towels left in the lost-and-found. They won't match, but do you care?

11. Use the dishwasher sparingly. Most of the time dishwashers can be great timesavers. But they can also be money drainers. Wash dishes by hand when possible.

12. Windex. It is man's favorite cheapskate substance. This one's the boss, the man, the big daddy, and the godfather of all cleaners. We like quick results and Windex does the trick. It's why we relate so well with the father in the movie *My Big Fat Greek Wedding*. He knew what guys all know: Windex cleans all surfaces, glass, appliances, kitchen table, and dusts off molding, It cleans automobile, seats, wheel rims and dashboards. It also kills aphids in your rose garden. If you were to buy just one quart of Windex to clean your counters, faucets, tabletops, window sills, glass, stove, floors and sinks, you would be cutting out expensive (and toxic) chemicals that would do the same task. Too bad they don't make a holster for it so you can carry that bad boy around on your hip.

13. The magic of baking soda - now you're talking. This is some great stuff. You can cook with it and you can eat it. You can clean stuff with it, and you can do your laundry with it. It keeps the fridge and your garbage disposal from smelling and you can sprinkle a little in your shoes as a deodorizer. You can brush your teeth with it, use it as underarm deodorant, you can wash your face with it and remove oily skin, and if you have halitosis (dog breath) you can gargle with it. It also cleans bathroom grout.

14. When ordering lunch at your favorite drive-through, order the kids meal and eat it yourself. There's just enough food to keep your weight down. Besides, how many retirees do you know who can handle a supersized anything?

15. At dinner gatherings, don't be shy about accepting leftovers to take home. (Just return the pan.)

16. Separate your loaf of bread into slices of four, place them in Ziploc bags and store them in the freezer. Bread spoils easily. This way you can take out and thaw only what you need.

17. If you're a single retiree, use "free dinner" coupons only on your second or third date. (Jeez!)

18. Sneak your own snacks into a movie theatre or ball game.

19. When vacationing, don't stay at hotels. Stay with family if they live in the same city you are visiting. Just don't overstay. House guests, like fish, smell after three days.

20. Wash out and reuse Ziploc bags. (Except the ones used for storing meat...for obvious reasons.)

WHAT IF THIS FRUGALISTA LIFESTYLE CATCHES ON?

Welcome to the *Buddhahood*. I hope you had as much fun reading this as I had writing it. What if the frugalista lifestyle catches on? And why shouldn't it? It's not difficult living the frugalista lifestyle. After all, it takes much more time and effort to be a trend-following, possession-hoarding worker bee than it does to follow your dream of being free to do the things you love. Maybe you are already there, retired and pleased with how your life is going, and you still found the book interesting. Or, you are still trying to figure out what to do next to make your life more satisfying. Either way, I hope you found a few nuggets of wisdom that helped add a little meaning or direction to your retirement journey. Whatever effect living a frugal, Zen lifestyle has on you, I know it will be a positive one.

Remember and use what I've taught you: Let the present embrace you. Always strive to get the most out of life that you possibly can. Keep an open mind and a closed wallet. Be yourself and do what you can with what you have, wherever you are. Then you'll be truly living Zen.

I love you, man!

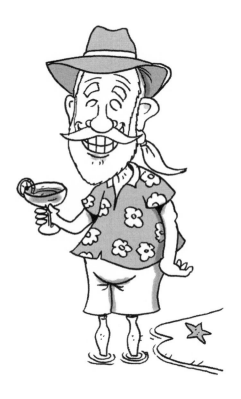

CREDIT WHERE CREDIT IS DUE

The golden rule requires that if a program inspires me, I should share it with other people who may like it as well. I am especially grateful to Richard Stallman for his inspiration and his e-book *Zen to Done*. But more so, for freely granting full permission to use some great tips and philosophies found in his *OpenSourceBlogging.com*

No retiree should go without keeping an arsenal such as I have listed for you below. Want to save a lot of cash? Then invest a little cash.

Written inspiration:

- Mel Ash: *"What Is Zen?"* Article from, Inner Self Magazine, August, 1999.
- Angela Anis Nin, Writer/poet
- William Bridges: *Transitions*
- Elisabeth Coleman: *"A Friend Stopped by."* PISS Post-Institutional Stress Syndrome.
- Brenda Shoshanna: *Zen And the Art of Love.*
- Melody Beattie: *The Language of Letting Go.*
- Ayn Rand: *Atlas Shrugged*, 1957.
- Elizabeth Barrett Browning: *Biography and Works.*

- Karen Salmansohn: *Ballsy: 99 Ways To Grow A Bigger Pair*.
- Leo Babauta: *www.Zen Habits.net*
- Gary R. McClain, Ph.D. and Eve Adamson: *Zen Living*.
- Patricia Evans: *The Verbally Abusive Relationship*.
- Mary Lloyd: *Super-Charged Retirement*.
- Richard Stallman: *Zen to Done*.
- Career Connection: Employment Newsletter, Minnesota, USA
- Dean Sluyter: *The Zen Commandments*; *Why the Chicken Crossed the Road and Other Hidden Enlightenment Teachings*.
- Wayne W. Dyer: *Your Erroneous Zones*.
- Cindy Heller: Ezine Articles
- Allen Klein: *Zen Humor: From Ah ha to Ha Ha!*
- Jeff Yeager: *The Ultimate Cheapskate*
- Robin Herbst & Julie Miller: *The Cheap Book*
- Mary Hunt: *The Complete Cheapskate*.
- Mark Miller: *The Complete Idiot's Guide to Being a Cheapskate*.
- Robert Kiyosaki: *Rich Dad, Poor Dad*.
- Andrew John & Stephen Blake: *Are You a Miserable Old Bastard?*
- Amy Dacyczyn: *The Complete Tightwad Gazette*.
- Ernie Zelinski: *How to Retire Happy, Wild and Free*.
- Dennis Waitley: *The Psychology of Winning*.
- Christina Brown: *Northern Cheapskate Website: www.northerncheapskate.com*
- David McKenna: *Retirement Is Not For Sissies*.
- Steve Pavlina: *Personal Development for Smart People*.
- Franz Metcalf: *What Would Buddha Do?*
- *The Grateful Dead: Rock Group*

-Fin-

ABOUT THE AUTHOR

Dr. Louis Gonzales is a retired educator and former CEO of several non-for-profit urban organizations in the Southwest and Midwest where as a seasoned, results-oriented manager, coach and educational consultant, developed great strategies for getting the most out of limited financial resources. Dr. Lou integrates his streetwise frugal skills with his psychology and Zen philosophy to successfully translate much of he has learned from the public and private sectors into similarly effective principles for men coming to grips with retirement.

Dr. Lou attended the California State University where he received a B.A. in English and a Masters Degree in Counseling/Psychology. His extensive work in urban education earned him a Ph.D. from Columbia Pacific University which led him to open his own consulting company and speak nationally on topics relating to urban education and issues, management, and the plight facing the retiring baby-boomer. His colleagues know him as a bright, brash and witty streetwise educator who thrills at attacking today's complacent systems in honest and humorous ways.

Made in the USA
San Bernardino, CA
21 December 2015